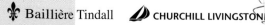

Dedicated to
Samuel Cade
Sorcha Heatlie
Wilar Than

Commissioning Editor: Ellen Green
Project Development Manager: Siân Jarman
Project Manager: Frances Affleck
Designer: Erik Bigland

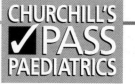

An Aid to the
MRCPCH
Viva

Second edition

Alan Cade
MBChB MRCP(UK) DCH MRCPCH
Lecturer in Paediatrics
Department of Paediatrics and Child Health
University of Leeds School of Medicine
Leeds, UK

Tracy Tinklin
BM MRCP(UK) MRCPCH
Consultant Paediatician
Derby Children's Hospital
Derby, UK

Donald Hodge
BSc(Hons) MBChB MRCP MRCPCH
Lecturer in Paediatrics and Child Health
The General Infirmary at Leeds
Leeds, UK

Foreword by

Professor Sir David Hull
FRCP Hon. FRCPCH Hon. FFPHM
Emeritus Professor of Child Health
Queen's Medical Centre
Nottingham, UK

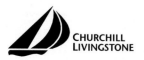

EDINBURGH LONDON NEW YORK PHILADELPHIA ST LOUIS SYDNEY TORONTO 2002

CHURCHILL LIVINGSTONE
An imprint of Harcourt Publishers Limited

© Harcourt Publishers Limited 2002

◢◢ is a registered trademark of Harcourt Publishers Limited

The rights of Alan Cade, Tracy Tinklin and Donald Hodge to be
identified as authors of this work have been asserted by them in
accordance with the Copyright, Designs and Patents Act 1988.

First edition 1995
Second edition 2002
ISBN 0-443-06494-6

British Library Cataloguing in Publication Data
A catalogue record for this book is available from the British Library.

Library of Congress Cataloging in Publication Data
A catalog record for this book is available from the Library of Congress.

Note
Medical knowledge is constantly changing. As new information
becomes available, changes in treatment, procedures, equipment and
the use of drugs become necessary. The authors and the publishers have
taken care to ensure that the information given in this text is accurate
and up to date. However, readers are strongly advised to confirm that
the information, especially with regard to drug usage, complies with the
latest legislation and standards of practice.

The
publisher's
policy is to use
**paper manufactured
from sustainable forest**

Printed in China

Foreword

The aim of this second edition, like the first, is to help candidates in the paediatric membership examination to perform well in the viva. Topics discussed in vivas continually change for they centre on current practice, new developments and present controversies. So it is essential for this 'Aid' to be rewritten at frequent intervals. That requires an extensive review and this is what the authors have done and they have done it well.

Again the content is determined by what questions candidates have been asked in recent years. The questions are posed in general categories and 'model' answers given. Each 'model' answer contains the essential information sprinkled with helpful suggestions and amusing asides. The recommendations are usually supported by reference to a key recent review or article. In preparing the answers the authors recognise that the candidate's knowledge will be incomplete and their understanding on some issues, somewhat fragile. In that situation it is not 'cheating' to adopt a strategy of damage limitation. The examiners are looking for judgement and an appreciation of the limits of clinical practice. Some examiners even ask questions to which they appreciate that the candidate cannot be expected to know the answer. There may not be an answer. Not knowing the answer and not being able to help are common experiences in practice! It is valid to explore how a candidate responds to such situations.

The book is attractive to look at and enjoyable to read. I would recommend it to any clinician that wishes to keep up to date in general paediatrics, particularly in areas beyond their speciality interest. It is a good way to see whether one is still up to speed. It can be read in bits, for example whilst awaiting the results of investigations or hoped for clinical improvement, or in lulls during committee or strategy meetings!

Perhaps examiners should read it. Then they would know what answers they can reasonably expect. Well, perhaps not. It might tempt them to spend their precious time thinking up new topics!

No examination is perfect, inevitably it will be unfair from time to time. The hope of the authors, which I share, is that this book will continue to reduce the chances of the careers of paediatricians in training being unreasonably delayed by this artificial but essential hurdle.

2001   David Hull

Preface to the Second Edition

It is now over five years since the first edition of the viva book was published. In that time the Part 2 membership clinical exam format has not changed at all. By contrast, there have been huge changes in the field of paediatrics. We now have our own Royal College; evidence-based medicine has been pushed to the fore; and molecular biology has revolutionised the diagnosis and management of many paediatric diseases. As paediatricians approaching the Part 2 viva, you are expected to keep up with both the information technology 'rat race' and increased expectations from well-informed and educated patients and parents (not to mention the membership examiner).

Many of the topics covered in the first edition have been dropped, not because they are no longer important, but simply because there are many new issues that warrant discussion. The subjects described are ones that have been asked during the last few years of examinations. First edition subjects that remain have been updated in the light of new developments. New subjects include recent advances and newer 'old chestnuts'. We have tried to maintain the format of a structured approach to questions, without overloading answers with huge amounts of facts. There is more than enough information in them to satisfy even the most well-informed examiner, although we have included references if further reading is preferred.

The best of luck with the viva — although we hope this book will reduce your dependence on it!

A.C.   T.T.   D.H.

Acknowledgements
Our thanks to Arun Shetty whose enthusiasm and persistence persuaded us to write the first edition. Personal and professional thanks to Peter Cooper for his great patience and overwhelming kindness - a true gentleman.

Contents

PASS

Contents

ix

INTRODUCTION

A paediatric MRCPCH candidate evolves from a very broad species but our research has revealed certain shared characteristics. He or she, though highly refined and intelligenced, is usually a very stressed animal, burdened by numerous evenings wiped-out by on-calls or their aftermath. There also appear to be two distinct subsets within the species. We have found a few individuals who hide themselves away with their objets d'art (a copy of *Forfar's* and a few piles of *Archives*) well in advance of the 2 months of torture. However, a second, much larger group (who are usually either fearful or suspicious of the first) seem to wake up one morning and discover that the turkey-shoot is only a couple of months away! This group then ponders the ensuing weeks in a daze of uncertainty, unsure of whether they should be spending their few remaining evenings attempting to drag an unsuspecting registrar or consultant around those all-too-infrequent 'hot-cases' or trying to chat up the hospital librarian. It is at this point that they usually start digging away at the shelves in their local medical bookshop, frantically clearing away the mountains of colourful gems intended for their spoiled adult MRCP cousins, in an attempt to uncover those rare paediatric nutshells.

We have tried to write a user-friendly guide that will lend itself both to systematic absorption and to frantic last-minute digestion and will therefore be of use to individuals from both of these subgroups. Our main aim is to provide the reader with a *system* that should maximise the marks obtained from the viva at whatever level of knowledge or experience he or she has attained. 'The viva system' is described in our opening section on viva principles and this will be built upon in the following chapters.

Our second (and less important) aim is to present framework factual answers to the commoner questions which arose from our survey of numerous examination candidates. We have divided these into sections so that the candidate may peruse a few topics in conjunction with his or her own formal preparation of that field.

Our answers are designed to provide an 'opening gambit' and it is important to realise that in the real viva the flowing candidate will usually be interrupted at frequent intervals. Some of our responses are written in a progressive question–answer style in order to simulate this. (We have used abbreviations for the sake of brevity; generally they should be avoided in the examination.)

From our own experiences, the viva (after the short cases) is the second most daunting component of the membership examination. It is also, all too frequently, neglected under the misapprehension that 'you can't fail on the viva alone'. This is not the case and one of us (having passed the other sections) was floored by a viva on statistics and epidemiology. In addition, it is usual to be borderline in at least one of the other sections (often the short cases) and the viva is an ideal opportunity to gain valuable, even life-saving, extra marks.

We hope this guide will be of use in the unsettling and often unsteady journey to the membership (and beyond) and it is for this purpose that it is primarily designed. However, it should also be of value to medical students and DCH candidates.

VIVA TECHNIQUE

Introduction

'... the viva was a terrifying ordeal. They can ask you anything so I didn't see any point in revising for it.'

It is true that, potentially, you may find yourself having a talk about anything that is in *Forfar's* or has ever been published in *Archives*. However, there are certain areas that are much more likely to crop up than others and we give a flavour of these in the main text of the book. It is not a bad thing to read the 'Medical Briefing' from the morning newspaper on the day of the exam. You might be surprised at how frequently the examiners obtain their viva questions from this as they travel to the examination centre.

More importantly, we believe that good viva technique can be learnt (no matter how nervous or disorganised in thought you feel you are). In the viva, it is not just what you say but how you say it that counts. We have conducted numerous mock vivas and it is apparent that certain candidates with a relatively superficial depth of knowledge can viva infinitely better than others with a thorough understanding, if armed with confidence and good technique.

We cannot stress enough that 3 or 4 hours spent in *mock vivas* (with any willing and motivated colleague) before the exam, practising what you glean from this book, will pay far more dividends than spending the equivalent time wading through obscure articles. (Although important, most candidates overestimate the required amount of journal experience.) Make these as formal as possible, including having two slightly hawkish 'examiners', a desk, a knock on the door and a priming, "I hope you had a smooth journey to London." Try it! After a while they can be quite enjoyable experiences for candidate and 'examiner' alike.

The viva format

During the clinical section of the membership examination you will encounter no less than six college examiners — two in the short cases, two in the long and two in the viva. The viva will last 20 minutes and will be conducted either in a quiet room or, occasionally, in a large hall. Though the latter is not ideal, most candidates usually say that you quickly become unaware of your surroundings.

One examiner will usually welcome you and may offer a handshake (do not offer yours first). You may be eased in with a social, "How was this morning?" Reply politely and avoid converting this into a long rambling chat. The examiners will then take 10 minutes each to bounce you around between different topics and test your mental agility. The other may well scribble away while you are in full flight. Do not be put off! This is normal. The first question will often be on a broad topic to ease you in gently and to allow your tongue to warm up. Try and settle down and relax during this time.

The College seems to use the viva to test areas that cannot readily be assessed in other parts of the examination. These are:

1. Emergency paediatrics
2. A referral (from a GP or hospital colleague)
3. Social paediatrics, ethics, epidemiology, statistics and management
4. Basic sciences (relevant to clinical practice)
5. Recent advances and contentious issues (the journals!)
6. Hunt the diagnosis ('What's in my mind?')

Above all, you must be solid and fluent when it comes to demonstrating your knowledge of emergency paediatrics.

You may also be asked a 'fun' question, often at the end of a viva. For example:

1. Tell me about an article that has changed your management.
2. What would you do with a research grant of £50 000?
3. Tell me about an important recent advance in the field of paediatrics.
4. How would you go about designing a neonatal unit?

The viva system

The examiner
There is no typical examiner. However, they are all practising paediatric consultants and are therefore, generally, a tamer breed than their adult cousins and should be amenable to a bit of charm. You will hear of 'hawks' and 'doves' and you should attempt to practise with colleagues from both species. You will probably find in reality that the examiner is in fact a 'mynah bird' and has the potential to resemble either species. Once practised, 'the system' can be used successfully to squeeze every last bit of 'doveishness' out of any hawk.

The candidate
On the day, you need to feel comfortable and confident and yet look smart and rather formal. Not easy!

Walk into the room confidently and smile when the examiners introduce themselves. Shake a pre-dried hand only when proffered. Speak with gentle confidence and avoid 'ums and ers'. We make no apologies for reiterating the importance of mock vivas. Sit straight! The examiner may well be in a bored slump in his or her chair. This is not an excuse to relax *your* attitude. Avoid attempts to simulate wild geese trying to take-off at the sight of a double-barrel . . .Keep flapping hands firmly under control on your lap.

Aggressive body language will be noticed. The viva is about the examiners liking you and feeling happy to trust you with the charge of children. Allow yourself to see both sides of an argument whilst still gently expressing your own opinion.

When all is said and done, thank the examiners (they are there for your sake) and leave quietly without slamming the door.

All ears

You will probably still be reeling from the dreaded short cases. Thoughts of " . . . if only I'd remembered to examine for radio–femoral delay" keep trying to well-up in your mind. It is easy to lose half of what the examiner says in the heat of the moment. Remember, the battle is not lost until the examination is over. Put what is done firmly out of your mind and concentrate hard on your two new examiners and your current task.

Simple consultation principles apply. Always make eye contact with the examiner who is quizzing you.

All about confidence

From our discussions with membership examiners, we cannot stress enough how important a *confident* manner is for successful negotiation into the College. It is difficult to come across as firm and decisive but not arrogant or over-dogmatic, yet this is what is called for. Treat the viva as an intelligent discussion with a consultant colleague rather than a formal interrogation.

Another approach is to pretend that you are a paediatric SHO talking to a group of third-year medical students. Even if your teaching contains the occasional factual error, you will still come across as someone who is competent in the medical care of small children. Again, numerous practice sessions will help to fine-tune your delivery style.

First impressions (your opening gambit)

There is more than a grain of truth in the adage, 'it is the first 2 minutes that count'. What you are essentially trying to do during the whole of the clinical section is to prove that you are a confident and sensible doctor and that you would be a fitting colleague in the examiner's own department. If you come across this way during those initial 'getting to know you' moments, you are much more likely to be forgiven for later ruffles.

Answer approach

1. *Start with definitions.* Keep things simple for as long as possible. On the whole, the membership viva is not a test of small-print, detailed knowledge. It is more a test of how you handle this knowledge and confirmation that you have a solid understanding of the principles of paediatrics.

   Where appropriate, start with well-accepted simple *definitions*. (It may help to carry around a notebook with definitions and opening gambits to the common paediatric topics.) These sound good and if you can switch to autopilot for a few seconds, you can use this time to plan the rest of your answer.

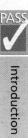

2. *Show flair.* You need to sound like your responses stem from experience and 'the counsel of years', not merely from textbooks. Show flair and style! The examiner will have had to endure numerous nervous candidates already that day and he is likely to be preoccupied by what his hotel has on the menu for dinner that evening. The more life you can instil into your 20 minutes, the more likely you are to eke precious marks from his thrifty nib.

'How would you manage a 4-year-old girl referred to your clinic with a history of urinary infections?'

Do not say:

> 'Well, eh, UTIs are quite an important problem in childhood and it is important to take a full history, carry out a thorough physical examination and then perform some investigations.'

This sounds boring and, quite frankly, a medical student could trot it out. It also sounds like you are talking *at* the examiner. Try:

> This is a common problem and one which I have had to deal with on many occasions in the clinic. I have come to realise that my first responsibility is to try and find out if these were genuine urinary infections as, if so, they can have far-reaching implications for a 4-year-old girl. Urinary infections in childhood may be of no real significance or they may indicate serious underlying disease where early discovery and intervention may prevent a lifetime of dealing with the dreadful spectre of chronic renal failure . . .

This sounds much more professional and should quickly convince the examiner that 'you know where he's coming from'. Note how the use of the first person 'I would' makes for an altogether more authoritative and interested response; using the second person produces a cold, depersonalised and somewhat boring answer.

3. *Cast-off wide.* Start with an overview of the subject and only then feed the examiners some detail.

4. *Structure your answers.* It is useful to *divide-up your response.* This not only provides structure to your answer, making it easier for the examiner to tune in to your thought processes, but it also makes you sound organised and in control.

'You are called to casualty to see a child who is fitting. What would your management be?'

> I would divide my management into: first, emergency procedures, including protecting the airway and controlling the fitting; and subsequently determining the cause of the seizures. Thus, on arrival in casualty, I would . . .

This division into emergency or early management, followed by subsequent management can be used to make you sound polished in a variety of other situations. There are countless other ways of dividing-up your answer and you should employ the technique of 'verbal headings' as much as possible. Scanty knowledge of a topic will sound much more voluminous and refined if what little there is, is classified!

5. *Common things first.* 'Common things are common, rare things are rare.' How often have you reeled this off to your medical students? Do not forget the principle when it comes to your own viva. When talking about erythema nodosum, make sure you talk about streptococcal and mycoplasmal infections before moving on to spout forth about the wonders of *Francisella tularensis*!

6. *Steer the conversation.* With practice and an agile sense of awareness of your *strengths* and *weaknesses*, you should be able to steer the examiner gently away from uncharted waters towards those you are more familiar with. Once you have settled into a question and demonstrated a sensible start, throw out the odd bit of bait. Occasionally an examiner will bite, in which case you have the opportunity to really impress.

For example, imagine you have been asked about the principles of the management of chronic renal failure, a topic on which you are a little shaky. However, you have recently read a good review article on erythropoietin. Not at the outset, but after having presented a confident opening gambit and demonstrated a bit of experience and flair, why not drop it into the conversation:

Anaemia in chronic renal failure is another important problem and its management has recently taken on a new lease of life since the introduction of genetically-engineered human erythropoietin.

The examiner, hopefully, will interrupt you with:

Ah, erythropoietin . . . that's expensive stuff. Tell us something about it.

7. *Avoid easy mistakes.* Avoid the dreaded 'I think'. Why not try an exercise where you sit in the examiner's chair and question a nervous friend. You will quickly see how little confidence is inspired when 'I think' precedes every sentence.

If you are not certain that a point you are going to make is absolutely accepted in paediatric practice, why not prefix it with 'I believe . . .'. This sounds more professional and comes across as opinion rather than uncertainty. (One of the functions of the viva is to show that you have formed sensible opinions in areas where the jury is still out.) Also, why not try, 'In my experience . . .'. It usually sounds great!

Do not open a can of worms. It is crass stupidity to mention hypophosphatasia if you know nothing about it. Having said that, you are not expected to be perfect and not even the examiner knows everything. You will make mistakes and also have virgin territory uncovered. Being comfortable handling what you do not know is just as important as handling what you do. Here are some examples:

My understanding of this rather difficult area is . . .
Of course, what I've said is nonsense. What I really mean is . . .

8. *Have fun.* Above all, try and use all your experience and training to allow you to have the confidence to enjoy yourself! If you do, the examiners are likely to as well, and your chances of being rewarded are multiplied.

Basic sciences and pathophysiology

1

DIFFERENTIATION OF THE GONADS

Q. What can you tell me about the factors governing sexual differentiation in the fetus?

Chromosomal sex is established at fertilisation. The Y chromosome contains the 'sex determining region' or SRY gene. If the SRY gene is present the bipotential gonad develops into a testis; if absent, an ovary is formed.

In the male fetus the testis is initially stimulated to produce testosterone by placental human chorionic gonadotrophin. Later, the fetal pituitary produces gonadotrophins. Production of testosterone stimulates the Wolffian ducts to form the epididymis, vas deferens and seminal vesicles. Testosterone is also converted by $5\text{-}\alpha\text{-reductase}$ to dihydrotestosterone, which promotes the development of the external genitalia.

In addition to testosterone, the fetal testis produces anti-Müllerian hormone, whose main role is to cause regression of the Müllerian ducts. It also prevents conversion of testosterone to estradiol and allows descent of the testes.

In the female fetus, there is no production of testosterone by the gonad so the Wolffian ducts regress. Since there is also no anti-Müllerian hormone, the Müllerian ducts are retained and develop into the female internal organs.

Q. Can you give any examples where the differentiation fails, leading to ambiguous genitalia?

In congenital adrenal hyperplasia, the excess fetal androgens in females cause virilisation of the external genitalia, leading to clitoral hypertrophy. However, since there is no testis producing anti-Müllerian hormone, the uterus and internal organs are present.

In complete androgen insensitivity, which may be caused by a receptor defect, a genotypically male child is unable to respond to testosterone or dihy-

9

drotestosterone and will have female external genitalia. However, the testes will have produced anti-Müllerian hormone so the Müllerian structures (i.e. uterus and fallopian tubes) will not be present. The diagnosis may not be made until puberty, when pubic or axillary hair fails to develop due to end-organ resistance to androgens.

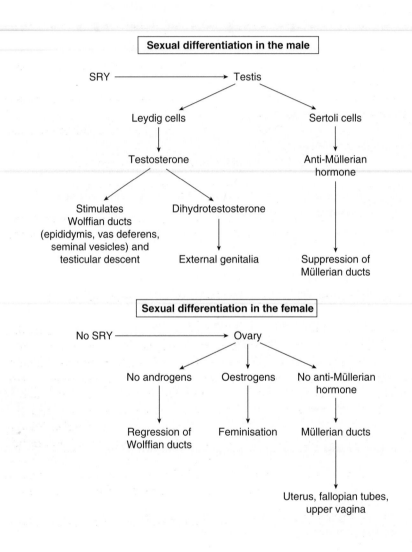

Sexual differentiation in the male

SRY ⟶ Testis

Leydig cells   Sertoli cells

Testosterone   Anti-Müllerian hormone

Stimulates Wolffian ducts (epididymis, vas deferens, seminal vesicles) and testicular descent

Dihydrotestosterone

External genitalia   Suppression of Müllerian ducts

Sexual differentiation in the female

No SRY ⟶ Ovary

No androgens   Oestrogens   No anti-Müllerian hormone

Regression of Wolffian ducts   Feminisation   Müllerian ducts

Uterus, fallopian tubes, upper vagina

IMMUNOMODULATION

Q. What do you understand by immunomodulation?

The immune system can be manipulated or modulated using two main methods — immunosuppression and immunopotentiation. I will deal with each of these in turn.

Immunosuppression is principally used to prevent rejection after organ transplantation. Four major groups of drugs are used:

1. *Corticosteroids* that alter the immune system principally by acting on 'resting macrophages' to reduce cell function;
2. *Purine synthesis* inhibitors, e.g. *azathioprine*, which act to inhibit proliferation of lymphocytes;
3. *Drugs* that alkylate DNA and inhibit lymphocyte proliferation, e.g. *cyclophosphamide*; and
4. Naturally occurring fungal metabolites, such as *cyclosporin*.

It must be remembered that all immunosuppressed children are at increased risk of infection.

Potentiation of the immune system is best achieved by vaccination but recently other drugs have become available, including the interferons and interleukin-2.

Q. You mentioned cyclosporin. Tell me a bit more about it.

Cyclosporin is a cyclic hydrophobic decapeptide. It is used as a first-line immunosuppressive agent in solid-organ transplantation. It acts to inhibit CD4+ cell-dependent proliferative responses by inhibiting the production of IL-2. It has variable oral absorption but this has been improved by the microemulsion formulation, Neoral. It is protein-bound in the circulation and is cleared by the liver. It enters cells by passive diffusion and binds to the intracellular receptor cyclophilin. The cyclosporin-cyclophilin complex inhibits calcineurin, an essential enzyme needed for the translocation of transcription factors to the cell nucleus. This inhibits gene transcription for interleukin-2. Cyclosporin has numerous side-effects, including nephrotoxicity, tremor, and hepatotoxicity. There are also numerous cosmetic side-effects, including hirsuitism and gingival hypertrophy.

It is essential that drug levels are monitored regularly and the dose adjusted accordingly.

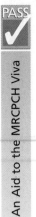
APOTOSIS

Q. What do you understand by the term 'apoptosis'?

Apoptosis is the name given to the process of natural, physiological cell death. It is different from cell death due to toxins and hypoxia, and *affects single cells in normal tissue*. Neighbouring cells move together to fill the space left by the dead cell. Apoptosis plays an essential role in the embryo for organ development and in the adult for maintenance of organ size.

Q. Do you know anything about the control of apoptosis?

It is believed that all living cells have the ability to undergo apoptosis, although many of the mechanisms initiating the process are still poorly understood. Factors known to induce apoptosis include free radicals, ultra-violet light, and deprivation/loss of essential hormones (e.g. the removal of oestrogen and progesterone which results in shedding of the endometrium — menstruation). In addition, numerous cellular receptors are able to mediate apoptosis, such as tumour necrosis factor and the Fas ligand. Many genes have been identified that are involved in the process of apoptosis, including the *BCL2* family, cytochrome C and tumour suppressor genes, *P53* and *P21*.

Cell destruction occurs as a result of activation of proteolytic enzymes. These are called *execution caspases* and effect apoptosis by destroying the cell cytoskeleton and fragmenting the DNA. This results in the formation of apoptotic bodies containing intracellular organelles that are subsequently taken up by phagocytic cells.

Q. How is apoptosis involved in disease processes?

Disease may occur in situations where there is too much apoptosis (e.g. in spinal muscular atrophy, where there is loss of neurons) or in situations where there is defective apoptosis and failure of removal of abnormal cells (cancers). Mutations in the *P53* tumour suppressor gene are believed to be responsible for a large proportion of human cancers.

REFERENCES
Afford S et al 2000 Demystified: apoptosis. Mol Pathol 53: 55–63

NITRIC OXIDE

Q. Tell me about nitric oxide.

Nitric oxide (NO) is synthesised by a variety of cell types within the body and is involved in a wide range of physiological and pathophysiological processes. For example: it is produced by the brain and is required for memory and learning; it is produced by the vascular endothelium to cause vasodilatation; and it is involved in the inflammatory response to inhibit leucocyte activation. Pathophysiologically, it has been implicated in atherosclerosis, pregnancy-induced hypertension and necrotising enterocolitis in preterm infants.

Q. Do you know how it is produced and excreted?

Endogenous NO (eNO) is produced from L-arginine, a semi-essential amino acid. The enzyme NO synthetase (NOS) is involved and L-citrulline is a by-product of the reaction:

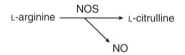

NO entering the bloodstream is rapidly bound with iron in haemoglobin, producing methaemoglobin. This is then rapidly converted back to haemoglobin and nitrate or nitrite. These nitrogen-containing compounds are then excreted by the kidneys. Because of the rapid metabolism of NO in the circulation it has no appreciable effect on systemic vascular resistance.

Inhaled NO (iNO), in theory, produces pulmonary vasodilatation as it is absorbed through the alveoli into the pulmonary vasculature but not systemic vasodilatation, thereby giving it a distinct advantage over other vasodilators in the treatment of pulmonary hypertension. Also, because it is inhaled, the better ventilated areas of lung will receive preferential delivery of NO. The resultant vasodilatation will divert blood from non-ventilated areas towards these areas of effective ventilation. This should reduce both V/Q mismatch and right to left shunting.

Q. Good! Tell me about your experience of using NO therapeutically.

I have seen it used in a number of clinical situations, particularly in the NICU and, to a lesser extent, on the PICU. Our unit uses a starting dose of 20 ppm NO in *term* infants for persistent pulmonary hypertension of the newborn (PPHN). In my limited experience it seems to be idiosyncratic in its effect. I have seen dramatic improvements in oxygenation in some infants, particularly in those with primary PPHN when iNO has been used in combination with HFOV; in others it has been ineffective, for example some babies with congenital diaphragmatic hernia. Although not used in the units I have worked in, I understand that NO has been used in *premature* infants at lower doses (5 ppm) for respiratory distress syndrome. Its effect is unclear.

In PICU, NO has been tried in ARDS, again with limited results. A poor response may be because ARDS is a multifactorial disease (pulmonary oedema, lung injury, neutrophil accumulation, right ventricular failure etc.), rather than just pulmonary hypertension. Present data suggest that iNO improves oxygenation in the majority of patients but does not alter the long-term outcome.

Q. Are there any side-effects of NO administration?

It reduces platelet activation and aggregation, increasing the bleeding time. This raises the concern about intraventricular haemorrhage in preterm infants, although I understand this has not been shown in practice. As already mentioned, methaemoglobin is produced in the circulation and its levels must be monitored during administration of NO (consider reducing or stopping NO if metHb is > 3%). Other unwanted effects include a reduction in neutrophil adhesion and, possibly, surfactant inactivation. Nitric dioxide produced in the ventilator circuit is potentially carcinogenic and so effective scavenging precautions should be in place.

Q. Do you know of any other research interest in NO?

Respiratory paediatricians are interested in measuring endogenous production and excretion of NO in exhaled breath as a marker of lower airway inflammation. If serial measurements of NO production could be measured accurately it may be possible to predict the onset of an acute exacerbation of asthma, for example, before there is clinical or spirometric evidence of respiratory compromise. Unfortunately, the vast majority of NO in exhaled breath originates from the sinuses, thereby limiting the value of this technique.

Key points

▲ Nitric oxide has a role in both physiological and pathophysiological processes in the body.

▲ It can be used therapeutically to improve V/Q mismatch in lung disease and in the treatment of pulmonary hypertension.

▲ Potential side-effects include decreased platelet activation and aggregation, reduced neutrophil adhesion, and methaemoglobinaemia.

▲ Its role in the inflammatory response may enable its measurement to be used clinically in monitoring acute inflammation in the future.

Tip

● More has been written about nitric oxide in the last decade than about the royal family! You need to be fully *au fait* with the subject and talk about your *personal* experience of its use to demonstrate your competence with it.

REFERENCES

Bohn D 1999 Nitric oxide in acute hypoxic respiratory failure: from the bench to the bedside and back again. J Pediatr 134: 387–389

Kinsella J P, Abman S H 1999 Recent developments in inhaled nitric oxide therapy of the newborn. Curr Opin Pediatr 11: 121–125

Nelin L D, Hoffman G M 1998 The use of inhaled nitric oxide in a wide variety of clinical problems. Pediatr Clin N Am 45: 531–548

EMBRYOLOGY OF THE GASTROINTESTINAL TRACT

Q. Tell me about the embryonic development of the gastrointestinal tract.

The development of the gastrointestinal tract goes through six phases, 4 antenatally and 2 postnatally:

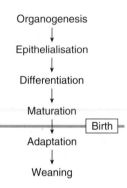

The primitive gut, formed from the endodermal layer of the embryonic disc, is first recognised as a tube from the 4th week after conception. During the next 36 weeks of intrauterine existence, the primitive gut elongates 1000-fold and by term measures approximately 4 m in length from mouth to anus. It can be divided into three sections, the foregut, midgut and hindgut, based on the blood supply to each section — coeliac axis, superior mesenteric, and inferior mesenteric arteries, respectively.

At 4 weeks, gastric and caecal swellings, pancreatic and liver buds and gallbladder are recognisable. By 6 weeks, the dorsal and ventral pancreatic buds have fused with 180° (rotation of the gut; the duodenum and splenic flexure of the large bowel are fixed; and further midgut rotation has commenced. Because of the rapid gut growth, the abdominal cavity cannot contain all the abdominal viscera and herniation of the intestine into the umbilical cord occurs by 7 weeks. Three weeks later, the gut returns to the expanded abdominal cavity and further differentiation over the next 10 weeks results in the defined anatomy of the newborn.

During the second half of gestation, further maturation results in identifiable digestive, absorptive and secretory functions, becoming increasingly complex in anticipation of extrauterine life.

Q. What is the difference between exomphalos and gastroschisis?

Exomphalos (omphalocele) occurs as a result of the failure of return of the normally herniated midgut around 10–12 weeks of gestation. At birth the gut (and sometimes other abdominal contents) are covered by peritoneum and amnion, arising from the umbilicus. Although it is not the case for all babies born with exomphalos, a significant proportion have associated anomalies, particularly renal and cardiac defects. It may also occur as part of a recognisable syndrome (Beckwith-Wiedemann syndrome) or chromosomal abnormality (Patau's and Edwards' syndromes).

Gastroschisis is the herniation of abdominal contents through a full-thickness defect in the anterior abdominal wall. In the majority of cases it is situated to the right of the umbilicus, which is normally formed. Because the gut is exposed in gastroschisis, it is important that minimal handling occurs preoperatively and that it is prevented from drying out by being wrapped in damp, warm gauze and clingfilm or put into specially designed bowel bags prior to urgent surgical intervention. Unlike exomphalos, gastroschisis is rarely associated with other anomalies, chromosomal abnormalities or syndromes. Its cause is unknown but the spontaneous involution of the right umbilical vein, causing a weakened area of the anterior abdominal wall has been postulated.

Exomphalos and gastroschisis are both detectable on antenatal ultrasound scanning. These infants can therefore be delivered in centres that offer paediatric surgical intervention. For both conditions, if the degree of herniated abdominal viscera is small, primary closure of the defect can be undertaken. If this is not possible, the creation of a silastic pouch (silo) and gradual reduction of the gut will allow closure of the anterior abdominal wall defect eventually. In some circumstances, the insertion of a Dakron patch may be necessary.

At delivery, bag and mask resuscitation should be avoided, instead proceeding to immediate intubation if it is necessary to offer respiratory support. A nasogastric tube should be inserted to deflate the stomach and/or prevent distension and i.v. fluids will be required. The insertion of a surgical central line at the time of operation allows the administration of total parenteral nutrition postoperatively — enteral feeds may not be tolerated for many weeks.

Key points

▲ The gut originates from the endodermal layer of the embryonic plate.

▲ The midgut hemiates into the amniotic sac by the 7th week and normally returns to the abdominal cavity by weeks 10–12.

▲ *Exomphalos* involves herniation through the umbilicus whereas *gastroschisis* is herniation through a full-thickness defect of the anterior abdominal wall (almost always on the right).

▲ Avoidance of bag and mask ventilation, the placement of a nasogastric tube, i.v. fluids, and antibiotics should be commenced soon after delivery in gastroschisis.

Tips

● Basic science questions are almost an inevitability in the viva. Included in this is embryology and although it may be years since you learnt it, a basic knowledge would be expected.

● Embryology of the gut is probably one of the easier systems to remember and, from our experience, the question most often asked. Remember, keep it simple.

● Explaining clearly the differences between exomphalos and gastroschisis demonstrates your hands-on experience of dealing with these relatively common neonatal surgical conditions. Babies with exomphalos warrant preoperative echocardiogram, renal ultrasound, and chromosomal studies to ensure that they do not have a lethal abnormality, whereas babies with gastroschisis need surgical intervention as soon as possible after delivery.

CELLULAR AND HUMORAL IMMUNITY

Q. Tell me about the differences between cell-mediated and humoral immunity.

To answer your question fully, I would like to start by explaining the basic make-up of the immune system and then move on to your specific question.

A primary purpose of the immune system is to distinguish between 'self' and 'non-self' and eliminate the latter by means of a number of different mechanisms — a process known as 'immunological surveillance'. Macrophages, monocytes, and dendritic cells, derived from stem cells in the bone marrow, are found throughout the body, including connective tissue, the airways and alveoli, the lymph nodes and the spleen. These cells act as antigen-presenting cells, digesting the antigen, breaking it down into peptide fragments and presenting processed antigen on their cell surfaces, bound with major histocompatibility complex class II molecules (human leucocyte antigen system).

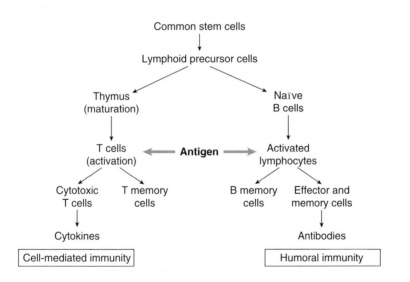

Both T and B cells express receptors on their cell surface that recognise specific antigenic material (*epitopes*) presented by the antigen-presenting cells (APCs). Coupling of the epitope on the APC with the T cell antigen receptor on the T lymphocytes leads to T cell proliferation and differentiation into activated T cells. These can then develop into:

— T helper cells (CD4+ subsets), which stimulate B cells and facilitate their transformation into plasma cells
— cytotoxic/effector T cells (CD8+ subsets), which go on to destroy antigen-containing cells, either directly or by cytokine release.

Cytokines are the collective term for a significant number of different proteins that are involved in cellular communication and include interleukins (IL), interferons (IFN), tissue necrosis factors, and granulocyte-macrophage colony-stimulating factor.

The T effector cell-mediated immune response

Antigenic binding to T cells results in the synthesis of interleukin-2 (IL-2). This protein stimulates the cloned expansion and differentiation of these antigen-specific T cells, which then act as cytotoxic cells. Once antigenic exposure ceases, the activated T cells cease their production of IL-2 and transform into resting cells (or 'memory' cells) in anticipation of future antigenic exposure.

The B cell-mediated immune response

Naïve B cells can combine with antigenic fragments on APCs directly by means of cell-surface immunoglobulins — a T cell-independent response. More usually, T cell/APC complexes combine with B cells expressing the same antigenic specificity — a T cell-dependent response. This causes B cell proliferation by clonal expansion and differentiation into antibody-producing cells. These mature cells produce the five classes of immunoglobulin, found in different sites around the body (IgA — mucous membranes; IgD — surface marker of virgin B cells; IgE — airways, gastrointestinal tract and lymph nodes; IgG — plasma; and IgM — intravascular).

Q. Tell me something about the differentiation of T helper cells and its relevance in the development of atopy.

Antigenic stimulation of the naïve T cell can result in the formation of two functional T helper lymphocyte subsets with different cytokine profiles. This is dependent on a number of factors:

— the nature of the antigen
— the timing of exposure to the antigen
— the genetic make-up (or atopic predisposition) of the individual

Typically, viral, bacterial, and protozoal antigens stimulate T helper 1 (Th1) cell production, whereas helminthic and 'allergenic' antigens stimulate T helper 2 (Th2) cell production. Interleukin-12 released from macrophages promotes Th1 cell differentiation, with subsequent IL-2 and IFNγ production. This results in a cell-mediated delayed-type hypersensitivity (type IV reaction). Allergens stimulate Th2 cell differentiation through the action of IL-4 with subsequent humoral immunity and IgE-mediated allergy (type I immediate reaction). Mast cell degeneration releases histamine and other mediators of the allergic response. Enhanced Th1 cell production inhibits Th2 cell differentiation and vice versa. Therefore, if it were possible to promote Th1 cell differentiation early in the programming of the immature immune system, or to switch off Th2 cell production in the mature immune system, it could be theoretically possible to prevent atopic disease.

At present it is not clear whether priming of the genetically predisposed immune system occurs in utero or in early extrauterine life. Immunomodulatory manoeuvres, such as avoidance of certain allergenic antigens in pregnancy, or the administration of specific immunomodulatory agents in early life, for example corticosteroids, may one day mean that respiratory paediatricians could be 'put out to graze'!

Key points

▲ Cell-mediated immunity = T cells, IL-2 and cytokines

▲ Humoral immunity = B cells and immunoglobulin production

▲ Bacterial, viral, and protozoal antigens = > Th1 production and IFNγ; allergenic, and helminthic antigens = > Th2 production and IgE

Tips

● Molecular biology has arrived and is here to stay. Hopefully the examiners you have are sufficiently 'long in the tooth' not to know much about it and therefore will not ask about it — but do not count on it!

● The controversies and research about the origins of atopy are an enormous field. This very simple introduction to the subject will hopefully see you through should you be asked about it all.

REFERENCE
Mackay I, Rosen F S 2000 The immune system. N Engl J Med 343: 108–117

BILIRUBIN METABOLISM

Q. Jaundice is a common problem in newborn infants. What can you tell us about the metabolism of bilirubin?

Bilirubin is the waste product of red blood cells and is normally excreted by the liver. Failure of excretion of bilirubin causes the clinical sign of jaundice which may also be caused by excessive bilirubin production.

Mature red blood cells have a lifespan of up to 120 days before being broken down, predominantly in the spleen, bone marrow, and liver. The released haemoglobin is phagocytosed by macrophages and broken into two parts — haem and globin. Other sources of haem include immature or defective red blood cells, myoglobin, and cytochromes. Iron is removed from the haem and transported for recycling by transferrin. The remaining product is biliverdin, which is rapidly reduced to unconjugated bilirubin by haem oxygenase.

Unconjugated bilirubin is carried to the liver bound to albumin. If unconjugated bilirubin is produced in excess of the available albumin it can pass into cells, as it is lipid-soluble. Passage into brain cells can cause damage, leading to *kernicterus*.

When unconjugated bilirubin reaches the liver, it is released from albumin and transfers across the easily permeable hepatocyte membrane to be bound to ligandin. This combination can be actively transported in the smooth endoplasmic reticulum, when conjugation takes place. Bilirubin is conjugated with glucuronic acid, by uridyl diphosphate glucuronyl transferase.

Once conjugated, bilirubin is actively secreted into the bile canaliculus when there is normal flow of bile acids from the hepatocytes. If the hepatocytes are damaged, bile cannot be excreted adequately and conjugated bilirubin builds up. After conjugation bilirubin is water-soluble so, in excess, it will pass into the urine from plasma. Since bilirubin is pigmented, the urine will be dark in colour.

This contrasts with unconjugated bilirubin, which is not water-soluble, so cannot pass into the urine. This means that urine is a normal colour in a jaundiced infant with unconjugated hyperbilirubinaemia.

Once conjugated bilirubin reaches the bile, it is excreted into the small intestine if the bile ducts are patent. It is hydrolysed by bacteria in the distal small intestine and large intestine to form stercobilinogen (also called faecal urobilinogen). Most of this is excreted in faeces after oxidisation to the pigment stercobilin. Pale stools are suggestive of biliary obstruction. A small proportion of stercobilinogen is absorbed into the portal circulation, where most is re-excreted into bile. However, a fraction escapes into the blood circulation and appears in the urine as urobilinogen. This means that small amounts of urobilinogen are detectable in normal urine, causing pigmentation of the urine which is particularly noticeable if the urine is concentrated.

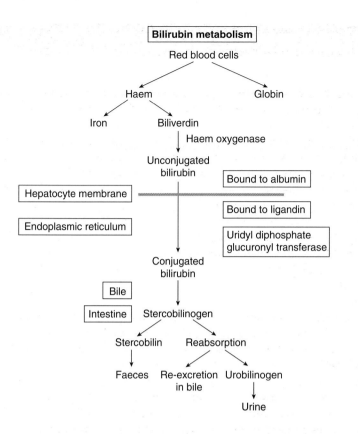

Bilirubin metabolism

Red blood cells

Haem   Globin

Iron   Biliverdin

Haem oxygenase

Unconjugated bilirubin

Bound to albumin

Hepatocyte membrane ———————————

Bound to ligandin

Endoplasmic reticulum

Uridyl diphosphate glucuronyl transferase

Conjugated bilirubin

Bile

Intestine   Stercobilinogen

Stercobilin   Reabsorption

Faeces   Re-excretion   Urobilinogen
          in bile

Urine

Q. So, with this in mind, what causes physiological jaundice in the infant?

Clinical jaundice may occur in a normal infant when the bilirubin level exceeds 85 µmol/L. It is considered to be physiological when no pathological cause is identified. Physiological jaundice occurs because the red blood cell load of a newborn infant is excess to requirement and blood cells are broken down rapidly during the first week of life, creating more haem, which is converted to bilirubin for excretion. The load of red cells is even higher when the infant has polycythaemia, which may be related to twin-to-twin transfusion, growth retardation, or delayed cord clamping. The neonatal liver is not fully matured and the enzyme systems are not sufficiently developed to cope with the high turnover of bilirubin.

Q. And what would cause you to be more concerned in a neonate with jaundice?

I would want to investigate jaundice further if the infant became jaundiced within 24 hours of birth, because this would suggest excessive haemolysis, or if the rate of rise of bilirubin were rapid. I would also be concerned if the infant had jaundice after 2 weeks, particularly if the urine was dark or the stools pale, as this suggests obstructive jaundice, which could be secondary to biliary atresia. I would obviously be concerned about any infant who seemed unwell in the presence of jaundice, since this might suggest sepsis or, less commonly, galactosaemia.

Key points

▲ Unconjugated bilirubin leads to kernicterus.

▲ Bilirubin is conjugated with glucuronic acid by uridyl diphosphate glucuronyl transferase.

▲ Excess conjugated bilirubin is water-soluble and causes dark urine in the jaundiced infant.

▲ Pale stools indicate biliary obstruction.

Tip

● The examiners have a list of suggested areas to cover and physiology is one of them. They also aim to ask about a neonatal issue, so bilirubin and jaundice are a good combination (see p. 88). When you are asked about physiology, try to relate it to your clinical knowledge as much as possible.

HAEMOGLOBIN AND THE OXYGEN DISSOCIATION CURVE

Q. What can you tell me about haemoglobin?

The haemoglobin molecule is made up of four subunits, each with a polypeptide chain (globin) and a haem group. The polypeptide chains occur in pairs and there are two types, α and β. Adult haemoglobin (HbA) is therefore denoted $\alpha_2\beta_2$. The haem group consists of an organic part, protoporphyrin, which is made up of four pyrrole groups in the so-called 'tetrapyrrole' ring, and an iron atom. The iron can be present in the ferrous (Fe^{2+}) or ferric (Fe^{3+}) form, although only the Fe^{2+} form can bind oxygen. Each haemoglobin molecule has 2,3-diphosphoglycerate (2,3-DPG) between its two β chains. Each haem can bind one molecule of oxygen — therefore one molecule of haemoglobin can transport four oxygen molecules

The binding of one oxygen molecule results in a destabilisation of the haemoglobin molecule, making it easier for the other three oxygen molecules to bind (*allosteric* properties). Therefore, the affinity for the fourth oxygen molecule is greater than for the first. This also works in reverse with liberation of the last oxygen molecule occurring far more easily than liberation of the first. This cooperative binding of oxygen allows haemoglobin to deliver twice as much oxygen and also explains the shape of the oxygen dissociation curve.

Q. Good, you mentioned the oxygen dissociation curve. What can you tell me about it?

The saturation of haemoglobin with oxygen depends on the tension of oxygen in the blood, pH, CO_2 tension, 2,3-DPG and temperature. A graph of percentage of saturation of haemoglobin by oxygen on the Y-axis against partial pressure of oxygen on the X-axis yields an S-shaped or *sigmoid curve*. This is due to the allosteric properties of the haemoglobin molecule. At low oxygen partial pressures, the binding of oxygen to haemoglobin is slow and therefore the curve is flat. The cooperative binding of oxygen is demonstrated by the steep part of the curve.

The affinity of haemoglobin for oxygen is decreased by an increase in CO_2 tension, increased H^+ concentration, increase in 2,3-DPG or an increase in temperature. This results in a shift of the curve to the right and therefore off-loading of oxygen from haemoglobin to the tissues. Oxygen is therefore delivered to where it is needed, as actively metabolising tissues produce H^+ and CO_2 and 2,3-DPG is formed from the metabolism of glucose in red blood cells. Without 2,3-DPG the curve would remain sigmoidal but displaced to the left. This means that haemoglobin saturation in the lungs would approach 100%, but little of this oxygen would be liberated when the blood arrives in the tissues.

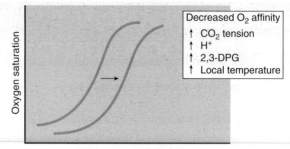

Oxygen pressure (pO_2)

Q. What do you know about fetal haemoglobin?

Fetal haemoglobin (HbF) contains two γ chains instead of the β chains seen in HbA and is therefore $\alpha_2\gamma_2$. HbF binds 2,3-DPG less strongly than HbA and therefore has a higher oxygen affinity. This means that, under physiological conditions, HbF is oxygenated at the expense of maternal HbA on the other side of the placenta.

CALCIUM METABOLISM

Q. Tell me something about calcium.

Calcium is an essential mineral and must be accumulated by the growing child. 99% of total body calcium is in bone with the remaining 1% present in various body fluids. Calcium has vital roles in cardiac and neuromuscular excitability, endocrine function, blood coagulation and enzymatic reactions.

Circulating calcium exists in two main forms. Around 50% of the total measured plasma calcium is freely ionised and it is this fraction that is biologically active and under homeostatic control. Another 40% is bound to protein (albumin) and is unavailable to the tissues. There is free exchange between these two groups. The remainder forms complexes with phosphate and other anions.

Various calculations are available to 'correct' calcium concentrations for abnormal albumin levels. A commonly used formula is to add 0.02 mmol/L for every 1 g/L the albumin is below 40 g/L. In situations where the serum albumin is high, 0.02 mmol/L is subtracted from the total plasma calcium for every 1 g/L above 48 g/L.

Calcium homeostasis is controlled by parathyroid hormone and 1,25-dihydroxycholecalciferol (which act to increase plasma calcium) and calcitonin (which acts to reduce plasma calcium).

Q. Tell me more about parathyroid hormone.

Parathyroid hormone (PTH) is the most important factor in controlling the level of free circulating ionised calcium. It is released by the four parathyroid glands in response to a fall in free calcium concentration and acts to increase the calcium levels by:

— stimulating osteoclasts, which release calcium and phosphate from bone;
— acting on distal renal tubules to promote calcium reabsorption and phosphate secretion;
— increasing gut absorption of calcium;
— stimulating renal synthesis of 1,25-dihydroxycholecalciferol.

The phosphaturic effect of PTH is not only physiologically important but an important action to bear in mind when it comes to understanding the pathophysiology of disorders of calcium metabolism.

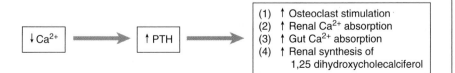

$\downarrow Ca^{2+}$ → $\uparrow PTH$ →
(1) $\uparrow$ Osteoclast stimulation
(2) $\uparrow$ Renal Ca^{2+} absorption
(3) $\uparrow$ Gut Ca^{2+} absorption
(4) $\uparrow$ Renal synthesis of 1,25 dihydroxycholecalciferol

Q. You mentioned 1,25–dihydroxycholecalciferol. What do you know about vitamin D and its metabolites?

Vitamin D refers to cholecalciferol (vitamin D_3). Vitamin D_3 is synthesised in the epidermis by the action of UV light on 7-dehydrocholesterol or is obtained from the diet. Vitamin D_3 is transported to the liver, bound to specific carrier proteins, where it is hydroxylated at the 25-position resulting in 25-hydroxy-D_3. It is then transported to the kidney where it is hydroxylated at the 1-position resulting in the active form, 1,25-dihydroxycholecalciferol (1,25–DHCC).

1,25-DHCC acts on intestinal cells of the gut and the kidneys to promote Ca^{2+} absorption. It also acts on bone (probably mediated by PTH) to mobilise calcium. In short-term homeostasis, the bone effects of PTH and 1,25-DHCC are the most important.

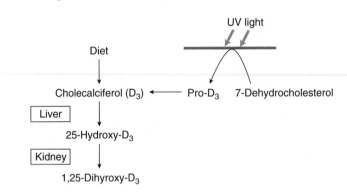

Q. Do you know anything about 24,25-dihydroxycholecalciferol?

Some of the 25-hydroxycholecalciferol at the kidney is hydroxylated at the 24- instead of the 1-position, yielding 24,25-dihydroxycholecalciferol. This has minimal activity compared to 1, 25-DHCC.

Q. Tell me about calcitonin.

Calcitonin is a hormone secreted by the parafollicular C cells of the thyroid gland. It is released in response to high plasma calcium. Its effects are opposite to those of PTH. It inhibits bone resorption and has calciuric and phosphaturic activity.

Its physiological importance as a hypocalcaemic hormone in the older child and adult is probably minor. Neither thyroidectomy nor calcitonin hypersecretion from medullary thyroid carcinoma affect plasma calcium levels. Calcitonin and 1,25-DHCC levels are higher in the fetus and infant although the importance of this is unexplained.

Q. What do you know about phosphate?

Phosphate (PO_4^{3-}) is an essential part of most biological systems, including nucleic acids. About 80% of all body phosphorus is in bone. Phosphate metabolism is very closely linked to calcium at a variety of levels, including mutual bonding in plasma and bone and their combined regulation by PTH and 1,25-DHCC. Unlike calcium, plasma inorganic phosphate concentration is age-related in childhood, declining from high levels in infancy.

RENAL PHYSIOLOGY

Q. What can you tell us about renal physiology?

The kidney's main function is to excrete waste products from the body while maintaining electrolyte and acid–base balance. It also has a role in producing renin, erythropoietin and Vitamin D. The kidneys are made up of *nephrons*, each containing a *glomerulus* through which fluid is filtered from the blood and a *tubule* in which the fluid is converted to urine by adjustment of the ultrafiltrate contents.

Fluid moves from the renal capillaries to the glomeruli by passive filtration, which depends on the higher hydrostatic pressure of the blood compared with the pressure in the lumen of the glomeruli. Large volumes of fluid pass through the kidney daily and although this passive process allows excretion of waste products such as urea and creatinine, both fluid and electrolytes then need to be reabsorbed in order to prevent dehydration and electrolyte depletion.

Reabsorption of fluid and electrolytes occurs in the renal tubules, leaving urine with an adjusted solute derived from the ultrafiltrate. The majority of sodium is reabsorbed in the proximal tubule. It diffuses passively from the tubular lumen into the tubular epithelial cell as a result of a negative potential in the cell. It is then transported actively out of the cell into the interstitium using energy produced by the cleavage of ATP. Potassium and hydrogen ions compete for secretion into the tubular lumen in exchange for sodium ions. Secretion of hydrogen ions into the urine controls acid–base balance.

Any remaining sodium in the solute passes to the distal nephron, where fine adjustments are made. When the level of circulating *aldosterone* is high, sodium is reabsorbed in exchange for potassium or hydrogen ions. The stimulus to aldosterone production in the adrenal gland comes from the production of *renin* in the kidney in response to reduced renal blood flow. Sodium retention in turn allows more water reabsorption, which restores low circulating blood volume.

Q. So, what governs the reabsorption of water in the kidney?

Water is reabsorbed passively along an osmotic gradient throughout the renal tubule, following sodium ions. The majority of water is reabsorbed in the proximal tubule with sodium ions, so the solute reaching the *loop of Henle* is reduced in volume, but is iso-osmotic. There is a counter-current mechanism operating in the loop of Henle which allows concentration or dilution of urine. Solute, in the form of sodium or chloride is pumped from the ascending loop to the descending loop, and water is freely absorbed from the descending loop. This means that the urine in the ascending loop is dilute, with the highest osmotic pressure at the tip of the loop and surrounding tissues of the medulla. In the presence of *antidiuretic hormone* (ADH), the walls of the distal tubule and collecting duct are permeable to water, allowing passive absorption of water along the osmotic gradient and concentration of urine. In the absence of ADH, for example if plasma is hypotonic, dilute urine is formed.

Q. Are there any differences between the adult kidney and the child's?

The term infant is born with a full complement of nephrons, but the glomerular filtration rate is reduced. Sodium absorption is well developed in the term infant, but the immature kidney of the preterm infant allows tubular sodium loss, with a resulting tendency to hyponatraemia.

Emergency paediatrics

2

DIABETIC KETOACIDOSIS

Q. What would you do with a ten-year-old girl brought in to the emergency department drowsy, breathless and unwell?

My first priority would be to ensure that the girl's airway was patent. I would introduce high-flow facial oxygen while establishing further history and undertaking my examination. I would ask whether the child had been previously well and whether there was a past history of asthma or diabetes mellitus in particular, or the possibility of drug ingestion, for example access to aspirin.

Q. Fine. The girl has been previously well until the last few weeks when she developed thirst and lethargy. How would you continue management?

I would confirm that the girl has diabetes mellitus by taking blood samples for glucose, urea and electrolytes, and bicarbonate or pH as I insert an intravenous line. While awaiting these results, I would check a blood sugar test stick. If this was high, I would continue to treat the girl for diabetic ketoacidosis.

Since the girl is clearly unwell, the most important therapeutic option is to provide intravenous fluids, as she is likely to be extremely dehydrated. I would start with 10 ml/kg of 0.9% saline to be given as quickly as possible. If her capillary return was sluggish, I would repeat this dose. I would then calculate a fluid replacement regime, replacing her maintenance fluids and calculated deficit over the next 24 to 36 hours. I would use clinical parameters such as heart rate and skin turgor to assess her level of dehydration, but I would not replace more than 10% of her body mass, as excessive rehydration can be dangerous. I would add potassium to the fluids unless there was a clear history of not passing urine, as the body deficit of potassium is usually considerable and hypokalaemia could be fatal.

I would insert a nasogastric tube if she had a reduced conscious level, as this might protect her from vomiting and consequent aspiration pneumonia.

Once the fluid regime is established I would start an insulin infusion at a constant rate, initially running at 0.1 units/kg/hour. The infusion rate should be slowed down if the blood sugar level is dropping by more than 5 mmol/L/hour, as a sudden change in blood sugar will cause a drop in osmolality. This may be a risk factor for one of the most serious complications of diabetic ketoacidosis, cerebral oedema.

Q. Interesting. Do you think that is the cause of cerebral oedema?

Well, the exact cause has not yet been clarified, but rapid rehydration and dropping plasma osmolality may well be contributing factors.

Q. How would cerebral oedema present?

In a fully conscious child, the initial warning sign may be a persistent headache; in a less responsive child a deterioration in conscious level may be the first sign. Either symptom should ring alarm bells, as there is a high mortality and morbidity from this condition. I would slow down fluid replacement and start a mannitol infusion (0.5 g/kg) immediately. Then, I would arrange a CT head scan and transfer her to an intensive care unit, where ventilation might be necessary.

ANAPHYLAXIS

Q. As the paediatric registrar, you have been called to casualty to see a 5-year-old boy who has been stung by a bee and has developed facial swelling and respiratory difficulties. Outline your management.

Anaphylaxis can be severe and life-threatening. Although most commonly seen after immunisation it is important not to forget that it may also be seen as a result of drugs, food (especially nuts) and insect stings.

My first priority would be the child's airway. As he already has respiratory difficulties, I would ensure that the paediatric anaesthetist is called and, in the meantime, I would administer 100% oxygen.

Only when I was happy with his airway and breathing would I then assess his circulation. I would want to obtain intravenous access but would first administer 0.5 ml 1 in 1000 deep i.m. adrenaline. If I were unable to obtain rapid intravenous access I would insert an intraosseous i.o. needle.

Access obtained, I would administer i.v./i.o. hydrocortisone 4 mg/kg and chlorpheniramine 0.2 mg/kg, assuming a weight of 18 kg, which is average for a 5-year-old. If the child's peripheral circulation was poor I would give colloid boluses of 20 ml/kg 4.5% human albumin solution.

If the child failed to respond I would administer intravenous adrenaline at a dose of 10 μg/kg, repeated every 15 minutes. If the child failed to respond to repeated boluses I would commence an adrenaline infusion at 0.1–5 μg/kg/minute.

Given the serious nature of this child's allergic response to a bee sting I would prescribe an adrenaline pen for his parents to have at home and teach

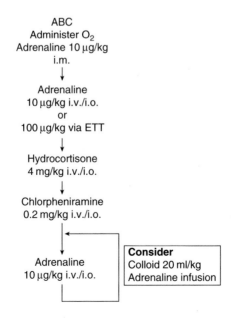

ABC
Administer O_2
Adrenaline 10 μg/kg
i.m.
↓
Adrenaline
10 μg/kg i.v./i.o.
or
100 μg/kg via ETT
↓
Hydrocortisone
4 mg/kg i.v./i.o.
↓
Chlorpheniramine
0.2 mg/kg i.v./i.o.
↓
Adrenaline
10 μg/kg i.v./i.o.

Consider
Colloid 20 ml/kg
Adrenaline infusion

them basic life support. The best treatment in anaphylaxis is allergen avoidance.

Q. You mentioned intraosseous needles. Tell me how to insert one.

The intraosseous route is a reliable and extremely valuable method of obtaining access to the vascular bed in critically ill young children. Absorption of drugs from the marrow space is rapid and similar to that from central venous access.

For a child under 2 years of age I would use a 16–20 gauge needle and for those over 2, a 12–16 gauge needle. I would insert the needle in the antero-medial surface of the proximal tibia, 2–3 cm distal to the tibial tuberosity to avoid the epiphyseal plate. I would take great care with asepsis to minimise the risk of osteomyelitis and would use local infiltration with lignocaine if the child was conscious. I would insert the needle at 90° to the skin and advance with a boring action through the cortex until I felt a loss of resistance.

In children over 5 years of age intraosseous needle insertion is difficult and it is preferable to obtain central access via a femoral, jugular, or subclavian vein.

Q. Good. What are the potential complications of this procedure?

Generally speaking, the procedure is safe and the benefits outweigh the risks in an emergency. However, osteomyelitis is an infrequent but well-recognised complication, with an incidence of <1%. Other complications include cellulitis, abscess formation, compartment syndrome, and pain. Other serious but thankfully rare complications include fat and bone marrow microemboli.

Tip

● As with all the paediatric emergencies, it is important that you can speak *confidently* about how you would handle the emergency situation.

REFERENCES
The Advanced Life Support Group 2001 Advanced paediatric life support — the practical approach. 3rd edn. BMJ Publishing Group
Kagy L, Blaiss M S 1998 Anaphylaxis in children. Pediatr Ann 27: 7–34

STATUS ASTHMATICUS

Q. How would you manage a child coming into hospital with an acute severe exacerbation of asthma?

In order to treat severe asthma it is obviously important to recognise the features of acute severe, and life-threatening asthma.

Table 3.1 Features of acute severe, and life threatening asthma

	Acute severe	*Life-threatening*
All children	Too breathless to talk Too breathless to feed	Agitation or decreased level of consciousness Fatigue or exhaustion Cyanosis, silent chest or poor respiratory effort
Children <5 years of age	Respiration $\geq$ 50 breaths per minute Pulse $\geq$ 140 beats per minute Use of accessory muscles	
Children 5–15 years of age	Respiration $\geq$ 40 breaths per minute Pulse $\geq$ 120 beats per minute PEF $\leq$ 50% predicted or best	

For all children, high-flow oxygen via a face mask should be given from arrival in hospital. Nebulised β_2-agonists should then be given as soon as possible after confirmation of the diagnosis by history and examination. If I felt that the child did have severe acute asthma I would give oral steroids at a dose of 1–2 mg/kg, up to a dose of 40 mg (20 mg for children aged 1–5 years). The onset of action of steroids is likely to be at least 4–5 hours and so the earlier they are given, the better. If the child has features of life-threatening asthma, i.v. hydrocortisone should be considered instead (100 mg 6-hourly for all ages). I would commence aminophylline with a loading dose of 5 mg/kg over 1 hour (unless the child was already on theophylline) followed by a maintenance infusion of 1 mg/kg/hour. A repeat dose of β_2-agonist can be mixed with ipratropium bromide.

If there is no improvement or clinical deterioration, oxygen and frequent nebulised β_2-agonists should be continued, together with 6-hourly ipratropium. All the while it is important to monitor oxygen saturation, keeping it above 92% with supplemental oxygen. The value of blood gas analysis is of little, if any, value in the immediate management of severe asthma. However, it is worthwhile measuring serum electrolytes to check potassium levels. I would perform a chest X-ray only if other diagnoses are suspected.

In some countries intravenous β_2-agonists are used more frequently than in the UK. Intravenous salbutamol is started in place of aminophylline for severe and life-threatening episodes at a loading dose of 15 µg/kg over 10 minutes, followed by an infusion of 1–5 µg/kg/minute.

Ongoing management of this child depends upon the response to treatment, but ideally should be continued in a high-dependency area. Fortunately, very few children will require intubation and ventilation — in these circumstances a skilled anaesthetist is required for induction of anaesthesia. There are several other therapies that have been used in intubated asthmatics, although I am not aware of any randomised controlled trials demonstrating their benefit:

— magnesium sulphate
— heliox
— glucagon
— calcium channel blockers
— clonidine

For children requiring admission to hospital because of acute severe, or life-threatening asthma a number of important issues should be in place prior to discharge:

— a 3–5 day (total) course of oral corticosteroids
— inhaler technique should have been checked
— they should have been on their discharge medication for at least 6 hours
— self medication/parental written instructions should be drawn up
— they should have a 1-week follow-up with the GP and with the paediatrician at 4 weeks post-discharge

These are recommendations from the 1995 review and position statement from the British Thoracic Society's *British guidelines on asthma management*.

Q. What about the management of chronic asthma?

This involves a stepwise approach to treatment, starting at a level appropriate to the severity of the disease and stepping down (or up) if and when control is achieved (or fails). For children over 5 and adults there are five steps of

Children over 5 years and adults

Step 1
Occasional use of relief bronchodilators

Step 2
Regular inhaled anti-inflammatory agents
● or cromoglycate, nedocromil or low dose inhaled steroids

Step 3
High dose inhaled steroids or low dose inhaled steroids plus long-acting β-agonists
● slow release theophylline, cromoglycate or nedocromil can be tried

Step 4
High dose inhaled steroids and regular bronchodilators
Plus
● slow release theophylline, or
● long-acting β-agonist (>5 years of age), or
● inhaled ipratropium or oxitropium, or
● cromoglycate or nedocromil

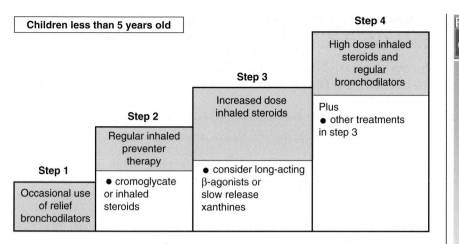

Children less than 5 years old

Step 1

Occasional use of relief bronchodilators

Step 2

Regular inhaled preventer therapy

- cromoglycate or inhaled steroids

Step 3

Increased dose inhaled steroids

- consider long-acting β-agonists or slow release xanthines

Step 4

High dose inhaled steroids and regular bronchodilators

Plus
- other treatments in step 3

treatment but for pre-school children, only four. The extra step in over-5s is the addition of regular single-dose oral steroids.

Great emphasis is placed on the correct administration of anti-asthma medication to maximise drug deposition within the lungs. Of particular importance is the use of large- and small- volume spacing devices for metered-dose inhalers. Other issues include the avoidance of provoking factors where possible, for example cigarette smoke, pets and damp, and the use of peak expiratory flow meters for older children to monitor response to treatment.

REFERENCE
British Thoracic Society 1997 British guidelines on asthma management: 1995 review and position statement. Thorax 52 (suppl. 1): S1–S24

STATUS EPILEPTICUS

Q. You are called to casualty to see a 4-year-old girl who has been fitting for 20 minutes. What would you do?

I would ensure that the girl was being given high-flow oxygen and go straight to casualty. A tonic-clonic seizure lasting for more than 10 minutes should be treated urgently. The complications of status epilepticus are usually due to hypoxia, so this must be avoided by adequate oxygenation.

I would quickly assess whether the girl has a patent airway. This is sometimes difficult during a seizure as the jaw may be clenched, but I would attempt to clear her airway of saliva with gentle suction and insert an oral airway. I would also tip her head back slightly and lift her chin forwards to help maintain her airway. I would give facial oxygen by high flow with a re-breathing circuit so that I was able to give close to 100% oxygen. This is important even if her oxygen saturations are good, because oxygen consumption is up to five times higher during status epilepticus.

I would assess the girl to confirm that she is having a convulsion, then arrange for her to have rectal diazepam if this had not already been given at home or in the ambulance. In the meantime, I would establish venous access and take blood to exclude hypoglycaemia and electrolyte abnormalities, such as hypocalcaemia. These should be corrected if present, as the convulsion will not respond to anticonvulsant drugs in the presence of hypocalcaemia.

Once venous access is established, I would give a dose of benzodiazepine intravenously. I have been used to giving diazepam intravenously, but it has been suggested that lorazepam might be more appropriate in status epilepticus because it has a longer duration of action.

While waiting for this first dose to have an effect, I would talk to the parents about their daughter if possible. After establishing the duration of the fit, I would ask whether she is known to have a seizure disorder and, if so, what anticonvulsants she is prescribed. If she has not previously had a convulsion, I would ask about current illnesses, particularly fever or any symptoms suggestive of meningitis. Febrile convulsions may occur in this age group and can be prolonged. I would also enquire about recent head injuries and look for signs of trauma. Finally, I would ask whether there were any medicines in the house which the girl might have taken.

If the girl does not stop fitting 10 minutes after the first dose of benzodiazepine, I would give a second dose. I would be reluctant to give more than two doses of benzodiazepine, as the risk of respiratory depression is increased after repeated doses. If the convulsion continues, I would give a dose of rectal paraldehyde mixed with an equal amount of oil. I have found this to be very effective and it can be used without risking further respiratory depression.

While waiting for the paraldehyde to take effect, I would prepare phenytoin at a dose of 18 mg/kg. I would give this after a further 10 minutes of convulsion, after establishing that the girl was not already on phenytoin. If she was, I would give phenobarbitone instead. I would ensure that the girl was on a cardiac monitor while giving the phenytoin over 20 minutes, as it can cause tachyarrhythmias. Once the phenytoin infusion had started, I would discuss the child with the intensive care unit as any further management would require intubation and ventilation with an induction of thiopentone. Even if the fitting had stopped at this stage, the girl is going to need close observation after a lengthy seizure such as this and I would prefer her to go to a high-dependency unit.

Once I was certain that seizure activity had stopped I would turn her onto her side as she is at risk of aspiration. I would arrange for appropriate investigations to be carried out if the cause of the fit was unknown.

Q. Thank you. You mentioned that lorazepam is now used in status epilepticus. Have you heard of any other benzodiazepines in use for seizures?

Yes. I understand that there have been some studies looking at the use of intranasal midazolam instead of rectal diazepam. It was used in a school for children with learning difficulties with a high rate of epilepsy, and seemed to be successful. However, that study involved only a small number of patients and I am not sure whether further work has confirmed the drug's effectiveness. It would certainly be an easy way of administering benzodiazepines if benefit can be proved.

REFERENCE
The Status Epilepticus Working Party 2000 The treatment of convulsive status epilepticus in children. Arch Dis Child 83: 415–419

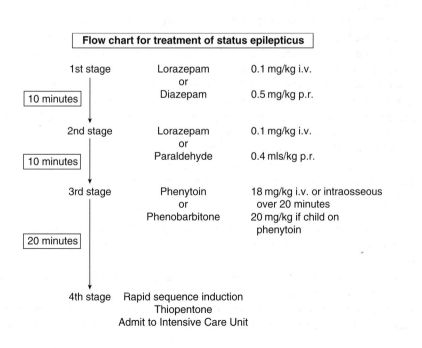

Flow chart for treatment of status epilepticus

1st stage	Lorazepam	0.1 mg/kg i.v.
	or	
10 minutes	Diazepam	0.5 mg/kg p.r.
2nd stage	Lorazepam	0.1 mg/kg i.v.
	or	
10 minutes	Paraldehyde	0.4 mls/kg p.r.
3rd stage	Phenytoin	18 mg/kg i.v. or intraosseous over 20 minutes
	or	
	Phenobarbitone	20 mg/kg if child on phenytoin
20 minutes		
4th stage	Rapid sequence induction Thiopentone Admit to Intensive Care Unit	

Emergency paediatrics

STRIDOR

Q. How would you manage a 3-year-old boy brought into the emergency department with stridor?

As with all emergencies, my priority would be to ensure that the boy has a patent airway, is breathing, and has an adequate circulation. I would be careful to avoid disturbing the boy at all, as distress might further compromise his airway. In an effort to gain the child's confidence, I would take a history from the mother while the child sits on her knee, with oxygen held in front of his face.

Although *epiglottitis* is rare since the introduction of immunisation against *Haemophilus influenza* type B, I would be looking for clues in the history which would help exclude epiglottitis. In particular, a history of a prodromal illness with cough, runny nose, and fever would suggest a viral cause for the stridor, while drooling or drowsiness in a child with sudden onset of stridor would alert me to the diagnosis of epiglottitis. *Acute laryngotracheitis* is the most common cause for acute stridor in this age group, but I would also want to exclude *bacterial tracheitis, allergic reaction*, and an *inhaled foreign body*.

On examination, I would look at the boy's posture: if he is sitting upright and still, particularly with head retraction in an effort to stabilise his airway, I would judge him to have severe stridor. If he was also pale, poorly perfused, and sweaty, I would be concerned that he has epiglottitis or bacterial tracheitis and would want to arrange for him to be intubated in a safe environment with experienced anaesthetists and ENT surgeons available.

Q. Your assessment suggests that the boy has viral croup.

I would assess the 'croup score', which gives an objective guide to the severity of the illness and allows comparison after treatment. The score includes the degree of stridor and recession, air entry into the chest, colour or oxygen saturation levels, and level of consciousness.

If the child has severe stridor, particularly if causing disturbed conscious level or desaturation, I would give 5 ml 1 in 1000 adrenaline solution by nebuliser, using oxygen. This should help to reduce the subglottic swelling, but usually only has a temporary effect. If severe stridor returns, the child might need transfer to the paediatric intensive care unit.

Q. What do you think of the role of steroids in the treatment of croup?

There is a growing body of evidence supporting the use of glucocorticoids in croup. They have been shown to reduce the admission rate and length of illness, as well as improving symptoms. A variety of steroids have been used, including nebulised budesonide, and intramuscular and oral dexamethasone.

In direct comparison with placebo, all of these have been shown to be beneficial, but there is no clear evidence to support one over another. Nebulised budesonide has theoretical advantages in that it reaches therapeutic levels quickly and has a low risk of systemic adverse effects because it is topical. However, serious adverse effects have not been shown with any of the preparations and dexamethasone is considerably cheaper, so it has been my practice to give a dose of oral dexamethasone to any child with moderate to severe croup after assessment shows that there is no suggestion of bacterial infection.

REFERENCE

Jaffe D M 1998 The treatment of croup with glucocorticoids. N Engl J Med 339: 553–554

THE SERIOUSLY INJURED CHILD

Q. Outline your management of a 4-year-old boy brought into A&E having been knocked down by a car at 40 mph.

This situation requires prompt action in order to maximise the child's opportunity for survival and prevent morbidity. Ideally, some warning of the child's arrival has been given so that the relevant medical and nursing staff are on standby. If this warning has not been given, I would call for extra help from senior colleagues when the child arrives.

There are four basic steps to assessment and management:

1. Initial assessment
2. Resuscitation
3. Secondary survey
4. Definitive care

Initial assessment

My initial assessment would be of the ABC of resuscitation. I would assess whether the child had a patent airway, while protecting the neck in case of cervical spine fracture. I would next assess his breathing before moving on to checking the circulation. I would assess the conscious level (using the Glasgow coma score) and pupillary reflexes.

Resuscitation

— **Airway** — I would perform a jaw thrust if needed, and not a head tilt. If there were any *obvious* foreign bodies in the mouth I would remove them (doing a 'blind' finger sweep of a child's mouth is not recommended as foreign bodies may be pushed further down the airway. If a foreign body is suspected it should be removed under direct vision)

— **Breathing** — If he did not have spontaneous and adequate respiration, intubation and ventilation would be necessary. I would seek the skills of a trained paediatric anaesthetist to perform the intubation unless urgent intubation were required

— **Circulation** — I would establish intravenous access rapidly but, if unsuccessful, insert an intraosseous needle. I would send blood for haematology, biochemistry and cross-matching. I would give appropriate intravenous/intraosseus fluids depending on the clinical situation

I would organise X-rays of the lateral cervical spine, chest and pelvis.

Secondary survey

Once I was happy that the child was stable, I would perform my secondary survey starting at the head, moving sequentially down to the feet. A thorough examination identifies potential problems that may require surgical or orthopaedic intervention. It is essential, meanwhile, that monitoring of vital signs is on-going and continuous. Once the child has had all the necessary investigations and has been seen by all the relevant specialities he would be ready for transfer to theatre or PICU.

THE UNCONSCIOUS CHILD

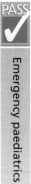
Q. You are called to see an unconscious 13-year-old girl in casualty. Run through your initial management of this problem.

On arrival in casualty, I would perform any life-saving manoeuvres that were necessary, going through the ABC of resuscitation. If the girl was breathing spontaneously with a patent airway, I would start high-flow oxygen while continuing my assessment. I would record a Glasgow coma score and if this was less than 8, I would arrange for intubation, as the child is unlikely to be able to protect her airway and is at risk of aspiration. I would ensure that we monitor the girl's heart rate, respiratory rate, saturations and blood pressure. I would also arrange for a blood sugar to be measured and give 5 ml/kg 10% dextrose i.v. if found to be low, followed by maintenance fluids which include dextrose.

Once stable, I would hope to obtain a history from an accompanying relative or friend, taking account of the findings of the ambulance crew. I would want to establish whether there had been any history of trauma or a previous history of epilepsy or diabetes mellitus. I would also want to know whether the girl had access to any drugs or alcohol.

During my examination, I would look for a 'Medic Alert' bracelet, which might tell me about diabetes, epilepsy or steroid treatment. A purpuric rash would be suggestive of meningococcal infection and skin pigmentation or nodules might be associated with epilepsy. I would look for signs of trauma, including the mouth, which might show signs of tongue-biting if she has had an epileptic convulsion. I would look for injection sites — either from insulin treatment or drug abuse. I would assess pupil size and function. Small pupils might suggest opiate poisoning; unequal pupils might indicate impending coning.

If I was still uncertain of the cause and treatment of choice, I would take blood for glucose, urea and electrolytes, liver function tests, white cell count and blood culture. I would consider doing an arterial blood gas and ammonia level, as well as taking samples for paracetamol and alcohol levels if this remained a concern. I would also collect urine for culture and toxicology. I would not want to do a lumbar puncture in an unconscious girl, but would certainly treat her with high-dose broad-spectrum antibiotics until I could exclude the diagnosis of meningitis or encephalitis.

If there was still no obvious cause for this girl's illness, I would arrange for a CT head scan as this might reveal signs of raised intracranial pressure, infection or intracranial haemorrhage.

Tip

● The emergency questions are vital! Make sure you know the up-to-date guidelines from the Advanced Paediatric Life Support Group.

MENINGOCOCCAL DISEASE

Q. Tell us about *Neisseria meningitidis*.

Neisseria meningitidis is a Gram-negative diplococcus that is carried in the nasopharynx of up to 10% of the asymptomatic healthy UK population. It is, however, the cause of most paediatric infectious disease deaths in the UK, resulting in approximately 250 childhood deaths a year from fulminant meningococcaemia and/or meningitis. It can produce one of four disease patterns:

1. Transient bacteraemia that resolves with no sequelae
2. Chronic meningococcaemia
3. Meningitis and invasion of other organs, e.g. joints, heart
4. Fulminant meningococcaemia

The clinical presentation depends on a number of factors, including: the age of the child (fulminant meningococcaemia is unusual under 6 months of age because of transference of maternal antibodies); the host's resistance factors (increased incidence in immunocompromised children); and the time between the onset of disease and presentation. Overcrowding and passive and active smoking are associated with an increased likelihood of disease.

Q. Tell us about the pathophysiology of meningococcal disease.

N. meningitidis crosses the epithelial lining of the nasopharynx and enters the bloodstream, where it multiplies. Coexistent viral infection may alter the integrity of the nasopharyngeal mucosa, explaining the common scenario of non-specific URTI symptoms for a few days prior to rapid deterioration. The multiplying organisms continually shed blebs from their outer membrane which contain lipopolysaccharides (endotoxin). *Endotoxin* stimulates the release of *pro-inflammatory mediators* from macrophages, monocytes, and endothelial cells. These key mediators are tumour necrosis factor alpha (TNFα) and interleukin-1 beta (IL-1β) and they exert a number of effects within the circulation:

— release of other cytokines and mediators of the acute inflammatory response, including CRP, fibrinogen, IL-4, IL-8, IL- 10 and cyclo-oxygenase products
— activation of neutrophils
— adherence of leucocytes to the endothelial surface
— complement and coagulation cascade activation

Serum levels of the pro-inflammatory cytokines have been shown to be associated with the severity of disease and outcome, higher levels occurring in more serious disease. These cytokines are cleared rapidly from the blood, followed by a rise in counter-regulatory cytokines, including interleukin 1 receptor antagonist (IL-1Ra), IL-10 and TNFα receptors.

Activation of the coagulation cascade results in clotting factor consumption, fibrin deposition in the microvasculature with endothelial damage and the development of DIC, intravascular thrombosis, and haemorrhagic necrosis. There is a fall in levels of protein S, protein C and antithrombin III within the circulation.

Capillary leak results in dramatic intravascular volume depletion, compensatory vasoconstriction and tachycardia. Myocardial function is directly compromised by endotoxin and together with capillary leak, contributes to the profound hypotension seen in overwhelming sepsis. Poor peripheral perfusion leads to a metabolic acidosis (anaerobic respiration) and a compensatory hyperventilation in an attempt to blow off the excess CO_2. Oxygen requirements rise with the increased work of breathing.

Q. How, then, would you manage a child admitted with fulminant meningococcaemia, bearing in mind the pathophysiological changes you have described?

Early recognition and initiation of treatment is of critical importance and may alter the prognosis significantly. As for all paediatric emergencies, rapid assessment and application of the ABC of resuscitation are necessary in the shocked and obtunded child. On arrival, the child should be administered oxygen and the ABC status should be assessed, intravenous access should be gained, routine bloods and cultures taken, and intravenous fluids and antibiotics given. Because of the significant capillary leak seen in meningococcal disease, large volumes of fluid replacement may be necessary, given as 4.5% human albumin solution. In the first instance I would give 20 ml/kg body weight over 5 minutes and reassess the peripheral circulation. If the capillary refill time remains diminished, I would repeat the dose and, following this, consider 'elective' intubation and ventilation if there were no signs of improvement. Further boluses of fluid, up to and beyond the child's total blood volume, may be required and this increases the risk of pulmonary oedema.

My choice of antibiotics would be a third-generation cephalosporin until isolation and sensitivity of the organism was known (almost all *N. meningitidis* isolated are fully penicillin-sensitive). Inotropic support should be considered early in those with septicaemia and my choice of agent would depend on the nature of the intravenous access I have obtained. I would use dobutamine peripherally (10–20 µg/kg/minute) and noradrenaline or adrenaline centrally, the latter being most effective. On obtaining intravenous access I would send bloods for calcium, phosphate, magnesium, glucose (all of which can be low), electrolytes, FBC, blood cultures, coagulation screen and blood gas. An EDTA sample for meningococcal PCR is warranted if the diagnosis is in doubt. Correction of any electrolyte and haematological disturbances is then imperative. There are a number of other therapeutic options that may be considered:

a) Correction of the coagulopathy with FFP, cryoprecipitate, heparin
b) Correction of the metabolic acidosis with bicarbonate infusions

c) The administration of corticosteroids (proven benefit in *H. influenzae* and *S. pneumoniae* meningitis, but not in meningococcal disease)
d) The use of other experimental treatments:
— ECMO
— plasma exchange, haemofiltration
— prostacyclin infusion for gangrenous peripheries
— protein C, antithrombin III, tissue plasminogen activator, TNFα receptor 1 and IL-1Ra infusions

Many of these therapies are experimental and not of proven value in improving the prognosis in meningococcal disease.

There are a number of other issues that are of importance in management of this devastating condition:

— isolation of the organism to rationalise antibiotic use and for public health measures. Every attempt should be made to confirm the diagnosis by throat swab, skin scrapings, blood cultures, PCR
— chemoprophylaxis for the patient and close 'kissing' contacts
— management of raised intracranial pressure by the use of mannitol, diuretics, moderate hyperventilation

REFERENCES
Kennedy N J, Duncan A W 1996 Acute meningococcaemia: recent advances in management (with particular reference to children). Anaesth Intens Care 24: 197–216
de Kleijn E D, Hazelzet J A, Kornelise R F, de Groot R 1998 Pathophysiology of meningoccal sepsis in children. Eur J Pediatr 157: 869–880
Pollard A J, Britto J, Nadel S et al 1999 Emergency management of meningococcal disease. Arch Dis Child 80: 290–296
van Brakel M J M, van Vught A J, Gemke R J B J 2000 Pediatric risk of mortality (PRISM) score in meningococcal disease. Eur J Pediatr 159: 232–236

BASIC LIFE SUPPORT

Q. Tell me about basic life support.

Knowledge of the principles of basic life support should be universal to lay and medical personnel alike. This is because basic principles are all that may be necessary to prevent morbidity and death in many emergency situations. This is particularly true in paediatrics, where the primary cause of cardiore-spiratory arrest is almost always from hypoxia rather than from cardiac disease. Simple airway manoeuvres may well be sufficient to reinstate an adequate airway, breathing and circulation. No equipment and minimal training is necessary. Adequate training for everyone to give effective basic life support should be encouraged.

The **SAFE** approach should be used:

Shout for help
Approach with care
Free from danger
Evaluate ABC

Should there not be an effective airway, breathing or circulation, this flow diagram may help and is easily remembered:

SAFE approach
↓
Are you alright?
↓
Airway opening manoeuvres
↓
Look, listen, feel
↓
5 rescue breaths
↓
Check pulse
↓
Start CPR
↓ ←——— 20 x 5:1 CPR cycles
Call emergency services

Airway
Airway manoeuvres:

— head tilt
— chin lift
— jaw thrust

Head tilt and chin lift should not be done if there is a history of trauma or if the nature of the injury is unknown. Over-extension of the neck by excessive head tilt should be avoided, particularly in the infant. Similarly, the finger sweep technique to remove foreign bodies in the mouth should be avoided as this can exacerbate, or cause, further problems.

LOOK (for chest wall movement) ─────────────┐
LISTEN (for gas exchange via the mouth or nose) ─┤──── For airway patency
FEEL (for gaseous exchange) ─────────────────┘

Breathing

Breathing is assessed by the *work* of breathing (rate, chest wall expansion, noise and nature of breathing), and the adequacy and effectiveness of breathing (presence of cyanosis, auscultation of the chest).

If there is no evidence of breathing then I would carry out five slow rescue breaths (1 to 1.5 seconds) to achieve visible expansion of the chest.

Circulation

Adequacy of the circulation is assessed by feeling a central pulse for 10 seconds. The heart rate should be >60 per second in infants and children and >100 per second in neonates. Effectiveness of the circulation is assessed by the presence of cyanosis, warmth of the peripheries, and conscious level.

Cardiac compression:

1 finger-breadth below nipple line in infants
1 cm above the xiphisternum in small children (<8 years)
2 cm above the xiphisternum in larger children (>8 years)

If there is no palpable pulse I would undertake five cardiac compressions after the five initial rescue breaths. I would proceed from this with a cycle of five cardiac compressions to one rescue breath, repeating the cycle every 5 seconds, i.e. 20 cycles a minute.

Q. You have mentioned foreign bodies but not how they should be dealt with. What would you do if 'finger-sweeping' is not recommended?

Foreign body inhalation is not an uncommon cause of cardiorespiratory arrest in young children. Basic principles are as follows:

Infants — 5 back blows, followed by 5 chest thrusts
Children — 5 back blows, followed by 5 abdominal thrusts / Heimlich manoeuvres

I would avoid abdominal thrusts in infants because of the risk of abdominal trauma. These manoeuvres should only be undertaken if a foreign body is very likely and initial airway manoeuvres are unsuccessful in establishing a patent airway.

Q. Do you know the success rate of out-of-hospital resuscitations?

If a child arrives at hospital with cardiac arrest, survival to hospital discharge is less than 10%. Neurological impairment in survivors is almost inevitable. If a pulse is present on arrival, survival to discharge is nearer 50% and 50% of these will leave hospital with no residual neurological deficit.

Key points

▲ Use the **SAFE** approach

▲ Airway — look, listen, feel

▲ Breathing — work, adequacy and effectiveness

▲ Circulation — adequacy and effectiveness

▲ 5 rescue breaths, 5 cardiac compressions, and then a cycle of 5 compressions to 1 breath every 5 seconds

Tips

● You need to know basic life support and you need to be able to *demonstrate* that you know it. Do not be surprised if the examiners throw a mannequin at you and ask you to demonstrate your skills, in either the short cases or the viva.

● If you have not attended an APLS course then make sure you say that you are on the waiting list, if asked!

REFERENCES
The Advanced Life Support Group 2001 Advanced paediatric life support — the practical approach. 3rd edn BMJ Publishing Group
European Resuscitation Council (ERC) 1997 Guidelines for paediatric basic life support. Resuscitation 34: 115–127
Whyte S D Wyllie J P 1999 Paediatric basic life support: a practical assessment. Resuscitation 41: 153–157

ADVANCED PAEDIATRIC LIFE SUPPORT

Q. What equipment would you require in order to intubate a child?

Most importantly, a second and third pair of hands! If it is likely to be a difficult intubation I would seek the assistance of a paediatric anaesthetist, continuing effective bag and mask ventilation until they arrived.

ETT × 3 — one size above and below the size anticipated
laryngoscope × 2
bag and mask with oxygen
suction
Magill's forceps
pharyngeal airways — assorted sizes
introducers, bougies
means of holding the ETT in place once positioned correctly
stethoscope
drugs

Q. Would you use drugs for the intubation of a neonate?

This depends on the reason for the child requiring intubation. If a newborn baby requires immediate, unexpected intubation at delivery then I may proceed without administering drugs first (except oxygen!). If I had a second pair of hands, effective bag and mask ventilation was being given, and appropriate drugs were to hand, then I may give medication prior to intubation if the delay in drawing up the drugs was not going to compromise the baby's prognosis. If a baby was being intubated electively or semi-electively, then I would always give sedation and analgesia (+/- paralysis), just as I would for a child. Typically, I would use:

morphine 100 µg/kg
+ midazolam 100 µg/kg
+/- suxamethonium 2 mg/kg
+/- atropine 20 µg/kg

Q. Once you have an ETT in place, what drugs can you give via this route should intravenous access be a problem?

The drugs of resuscitation that can be given via this route are adrenaline, atropine, lidocaine (lignocaine), and oxygen. Dosages would be 2–3 × that normally given by the intravenous route (see above).

Q. You mention oxygen as one of the drugs of resuscitation. Do you know of any possible detrimental effects of using oxygen in resuscitation?

There are a number of possible reasons why using 100% oxygen in the resuscitation process may be less effective than using air. Resulting hyperoxaemia may lead to:

a) reduction in cerebral blood flow
b) increased oxygen free radical formation, leading to
   —↑ lipid peroxidation and cell membrane injury
   — induction of apoptosis
   — DNA damage
c) increased brain metabolism
d) increased inflammatory response

    The Resair 2 study, a multi-centre study involving over 600 babies in six countries, compared resuscitation with room air and with 100% oxygen in newborn infants >29 weeks gestation. This demonstrated a greater delay in time to first breath and time to first cry in those given 100% oxygen when compared with those given room air. It also demonstrated a non-significant decrease in mortality and hypoxic ischaemic encephalopathy (grades 2 and 3) in those given room air. The study concluded that for infants without lung pathology, room air may well be equally as effective (or more effective) than 100% oxygen. For those with lung pathology, for example meconium aspiration syndrome, higher oxygen concentrations than air are probably beneficial however.

    Until more randomised controlled studies of oxygen versus room air (or even lower concentrations of oxygen) have been undertaken, both in neonates and children, I would continue to use higher concentrations of oxygen in all resuscitation situations.

Notes

There are some useful formulae and dosages for APLS:

ETT diameter*	(Age / 4) + 4	
ETT length*	(Age / 2) + 12	orally intubated
	(Age / 2) + 15	nasally intubated
Weight* (kg)	(Age + 4) × 2	
Adrenaline dose	0.1 ml / kg 1:10 000, followed by 0.1 ml/kg 1:1000	
Atropine dosage	20µg/kg	
$NaHCO_3$	1–2 ml/kg 8.4% sodium bicarbonate, diluted	
10% dextrose	5 ml/kg	
Lidocaine (lignocaine) 1%	0.1 ml/kg (1 mg/kg)	
DC shock	2 J/kg, 2 J/kg, then 4 J/kg	

The formulae provide an easily remembered guide, although some can only be applied to children over 1 year of age*. A well organised assessment unit/emergency department should have resuscitation charts available for immediate confirmation of appropriate ET tube sizes, emergency drug dosages etc.

The choice of induction agents for intubating children is endless. All anaesthetists will have their own cocktail and tell you that they use their combination because "they feel comfortable with them". Very useful except to the uninformed paediatrician!

It is important to state that current opinion, based on available evidence, advises the use of drugs in the *elective* situation. A recent survey of neonatal units demonstrated a woeful underuse of agents for intubation. This is unacceptable, although the older examiners may never have used an induction agent in their neonatal clinical practice — so be careful how you phrase things! This discussion may then move forward to questioning whether a neonate has the ability to feel and appreciate pain. Work from Levene et al and Rutter et al in Leeds and Nottingham, respectively, should dispel any notion about the analgesic properties of prematurity.

Key points

▲ Drug dosages, routes of administration, and possible side-effects must be learnt.

▲ Induction agents for elective intubations should be used without exception for all age groups, including neonates.

▲ The benefits (or disadvantages) of using 100% oxygen over room air in the resuscitation situation are not clear.

Tip

● APLS skills must be second nature. It is unlikely that you will be asked to demonstrate these skills in the viva, but you never know!

REFERENCES

The Advanced Life Support Group 2001 Advanced paediatric life support — the practical approach. 3rd edn. BMJ Publishing Group

Saugstad O D 1998 Resuscitation with room-air or oxygen supplementation. Clinics Perinatol 25: 741–756

Saugstad O D, Rootwelt T, Aalen O 1998 Resuscitation of asphyxiated newborn infants with room-air or oxygen: an international controlled trial. The Resair 2 study. Pediatrics 102: e1

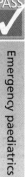

POISONING

Q. Tell me about poisoning in children.

There are two peaks in the incidence of poisoning during childhood — *accidental poisoning* around the age of 2 years (when children are increasingly mobile and inquisitive) and then another during adolescence as a result of *deliberate ingestion*. Although around 45 000 children under the age of 5 years attend casualty departments every year in the UK with accidental poisoning, only a minority develop serious toxicity. In the majority, observation and simple supportive measures are all that is required. However, a small number of poisoned young children (and a higher proportion of adolescents) will have taken sufficient toxin, potentially, to cause harm.

As with any paediatric emergency, the ABC of resuscitation must be the first step in management. Drugs (and plants) have a number of common side-effects in overdosage:

1. *Respiratory depression*: inadequate respiratory effort requires O_2 saturation monitoring. Blood gas analysis may be helpful, and in more serious cases intubation and ventilatory support may be necessary.
2. *Hypotension and tachycardia* secondary to 'shock': intravenous fluids +/- inotropic support should be considered.
3. *CNS depression and convulsions*: treatment of convulsions is the same for poisoning as in other causes of convulsions.
4. *Acidosis*: correction with bicarbonate may be beneficial.

For all significant (or potentially significant) poisoning, *decontamination* should be carried out as early as possible after ingestion or exposure. This involves:

— prevention of further exposure: removal of contaminated clothing, cleaning the mouth or skin etc.
— decontamination: skin and eyes by irrigation, gut decontamination using a variety of measures

Q. Tell me about some of those measures.

There are four usual methods I am aware of:

1. Induction of emesis
2. Gastric lavage
3. Activated charcoal administration
4. Whole bowel irrigation

Up until a few years ago, the induction of emesis by the administration of ipecacuanha syrup was the usual action for most poisons. However, there has been a move away from this in favour of *activated charcoal*. Exceptions to this include the ingestion of acid, alkali, alcohols, glycols, metals, cyanide, iron and a few other poisons and drugs which are not absorbed (or poorly absorbed) by the activated charcoal. Other exceptions include those poisons for which the antidote is to be given by the enteral route, and the activated charcoal deactivates the antidote as well as the poison itself. For some ingestions, repeated doses of charcoal are necessary, for example salicylates, carbamazepine, phenytoin, theophylline, barbiturates and sustained-release preparations.

Gastric lavage is rarely used and must not be considered unless a child can effectively maintain their own airway (unless they are artificially ventilated with a cuffed endotracheal tube in place). One indication for gastric lavage, however, is iron poisoning because it is not absorbed by charcoal and it causes significant morbidity in overdosage.

Whole bowel irrigation, using polyethylene glycol-electrolyte solution (e.g. Klean-Prep) in doses of 15–40 ml/kg/hour, is continued until the rectal effluent resembles the solution being given at the 'top end' and is useful for poisoning with iron and sustained-release preparations.

There are a number of other methods of active drug elimination from the body, including haemodialysis, haemofiltration, plasmapheresis and plasma exchange. The need for these in paediatric poisoning is rare.

Q. What about investigations in cases of apparent or suspected poisoning?

Fortunately, the number of deaths from poisoning in the under-5s per year is extremely low (between two and ten per annum). Sadly, between one and five deaths a year are due to ingestion deliberately initiated by another person (Münchhausen syndrome by proxy). For many young children admitted with symptoms and signs that do not fit a specific clinical picture, poisoning (either deliberate or accidental) *must* be considered.

If it is known (or suspected) that the child has taken aspirin, paracetamol, iron, methanol, ethylene glycol, heavy metals, or lithium, then measurement of serum levels is necessary to gauge the severity of overdosage and to monitor the effectiveness of treatment. As mentioned previously, blood gas analysis will assess the degree of metabolic acidosis in considering bicarbonate treatment and may help in the decision to artificially ventilate a child. Some agents induce renal and liver impairment and so electrolyte and liver function testing (including clotting factors) is justified. Some drugs (lead, iron and mercury) are radio-opaque and so abdominal X-rays may indicate whether ingestion has actually taken place and may be used to assess the effectiveness of gastric decontamination.

Q. Quickly tell us about iron poisoning in children.

Although iron overdosage is fairly common in children, serious poisoning is uncommon. Iron rapidly crosses the mucosal barrier of the stomach, entering the circulation, where it is bound to transferrin. In overdosage, transferrin becomes saturated and free iron is rapidly cleared by uptake into parenchymal cells. Here it causes mitochondrial damage and cell death. The liver parenchyma is particularly affected by iron overload, leading to hepatic failure, hypoglycaemia and coagulopathy.

The features of iron poisoning can be divided into four phases:

1. *30 minutes – 6 hours* post-ingestion: diarrhoea and vomiting, gastrointestinal haemorrhage/perforation, drowsiness, ↑ WCC, ↑ glucose.
2. *6–24 hours* post-ingestion: recovery or rapid passage to the next phase of poisoning.
3. *12–48 hours* post-ingestion: lethargy, coma, convulsions, renal and hepatic failure, gastrointestinal haemorrhage, pulmonary oedema, circulatory collapse.
4. *2–5 weeks*: gastrointestinal stricture formation.

I would be guided in my management by the advice obtained from the poisons centre, although treatment is determined to a great extent by the child's clinical condition and the serum iron concentrations (done at 4 hours post-ingestion or earlier if desferrioxamine is to be commenced). *Gut decontamination*, by gastric lavage or whole bowel irrigation, is necessary if ingestion is confirmed by abdominal X-ray or serum iron concentrations, or in any child with a high index of suspicion of significant ingestion. *Chelation therapy*, using desferrioxamine should be commenced immediately in symptomatic children, even if serum levels are unavailable. The dosage used is normally 15 mg/kg/hour and should be continued for up to 24 hours post-ingestion. For patients with shock, intravenous fluid replacement is required and regular monitoring of renal and hepatic function with appropriate intervention if indicated.

Tip

● It is impossible to know how to manage *every* type of poisoning in children. Indeed, you can reassure the examiners by stating that you would always phone the poisons centre for advice — they cannot criticise you for this cautious approach because it is always better to be safe than sorry! However, a basic knowledge of the principles is expected and knowledge of the specific treatments for iron, paracetamol and salicylate poisoning is advisable.

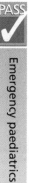

RESUSCITATION FLUIDS

Q. What would be your choice of fluid in the resuscitation of children?

That would depend mainly on the suspected cause of illness. For example, if the child had been involved in a road traffic accident, hypovolaemia secondary to blood loss is the most likely cause of the need for resuscitation, so I would prefer to use *whole blood* as volume replacement. Sometimes, it is necessary to use O negative blood after trauma but, where possible, I would want to use blood matched for the patient. If compatible blood was not readily available, it would be important to use a fluid which increases intravascular oncotic pressure and stays in the circulation for a reasonable period of time.

There has been controversy over which colloid is safe to use in children recently, following the publication of a systematic review of randomised controlled trials in the use of *albumin solutions*. This paper suggested that there was an increased mortality in patients treated with albumin solutions. However, few of the trials included in the review involved children or neonates. We tend to use fluids for resuscitation most commonly in children with sepsis syndromes, and only one trial included patients in this category. Although systematic reviews of randomised controlled trials are the gold standard for research, they must be treated with common sense and if the patient groups selected are not relevant to our own practice, the results can not be applied to that practice.

Paediatricians have generally had a lot of experience with the use of albumin solutions for the resuscitation of the septicaemic child and many centres would argue that aggressive fluid resuscitation improves prognosis in these children. While one should not rely on anecdote, there is no evidence and less experience supporting the use of other synthetic colloid solutions in children. *Synthetic solutions* are either gelatin-based or starch-based. Both carry a risk of anaphylactic reaction and gelatin solutions do not tend to stay in the intravascular compartment for much longer than *crystalloid solution*.

There is a theoretical risk of infection associated with the use of albumin solutions as they are derived from blood products, so it is important to avoid their use when possible. Personally, I prefer to use a 20 ml/kg bolus of 0.9% saline in the first instance for most children with hypovolaemia. However, if there is not a response to this crystalloid bolus, I would tend to follow with 10 ml/kg of 4.5% albumin solution.

REFERENCE
Cochrane Injuries Group Albumin Reviewers 1998 Human albumin administration in critically ill patients: systematic review of randomised controlled trials. B Med J 317: 235–240

MANAGEMENT OF BURNS

Q. What do you know about burns and scalds in children?

50 000 children attend casualty each year with burns and scalds. The majority of these are preventable, and public education via the media, GP waiting rooms, and health educators should be in place in order to minimise the risk of injuries. Most fatalities occur in house fires, with the most common cause of death being smoke inhalation rather than burns. There are three degrees of burns. *First-degree* burns involve the epithelium only and are red and painful, e.g. sunburn. *Second-degree* burns involve the epithelium and corneum, are red and painful, and blister. *Third-degree* (or full-thickness) burns involve the dermis and are white, charred and painless, and will result in scars.

Q. Outline your management of a 5-year-old brought into casualty with severe burns.

For a child attending casualty with significant burns there are a number of important areas in the emergency management. These are: ABC, history, fluid management, analgesia, and specific problems pertinent to the burns. I would like to discuss each of these in turn.

ABC

My first priority would be the child's airway, breathing and circulation; I would assess the burns as part of my secondary survey. I would ensure that the child has a patent airway and would examine the nose for evidence of soot and eyebrows for evidence of singeing — these may indicate smoke inhalation. I would administer 100% oxygen in all cases. If I suspected smoke inhalation, I would ask for the paediatric anaesthetist to be called as the child may develop laryngeal obstruction. I would then assess the breathing. Next, I would assess the circulation by looking at skin perfusion, pulse and blood pressure. I would establish intravenous or intraosseous access, and if the child had evidence of shock I would administer 20 ml/kg of colloid. While inserting a drip I would take blood for FBC, U&E, sugar, crossmatch, and carboxy-haemoglobin levels. If the child was still wearing hot clothes, I would remove them. If it was a chemical burn I would irrigate the burns immediately.

Once I was happy with the child's ABC I would proceed with my secondary survey: assessing the neurological state; looking for evidence of other injuries; and examination of the burns for extent and depth. The 'Wallace's rule of nines' cannot be used in children under 14 years of age and in these children a 'Lund and Browder chart' should be used, which takes into account the differential proportion of children's limbs. Alternatively, knowing that the palm of a child is proportional to 1% of body surface area, it can be used to estimate the total burn area. I would draw all the burn sites on a *burns chart* for documentation purposes and to avoid repeated re-examination.

History

I would try to gain as much information about the burn as possible from the ambulance crew or family. In particular, I would want to know the time of the burn (so that fluid replacement can be calculated from this time rather than from time of presentation), what has caused the burn (? chemical), and assess whether there is any chance of other injuries (? explosion). If the child has been involved in a house fire, I would enquire about where the child was found, in order to determine if smoke inhalation could be a potential problem.

Fluid management

Children with >10% burns will require maintenance intravenous fluids plus additional fluids, calculated using the following equation:

Additional fluid (ml) = % burn surface area × weight (kg) × 4

I would administer this as 4.5% human albumin solution and would give half of this volume over the first 8 hours after the burn occurred and the remainder over the next 16 hours. Fluid balance is critical to avoid organ dysfunction and children with significant burns should have a central line and a urinary catheter inserted.

Analgesia

The child may be in severe pain and I would use intravenous morphine for analgesia.

Burns management

I would clean the burns and cover them with sterile dressings. If the child had 10% secondary- and/or third-degree burns, >5% third-degree burns or burns to the face, mouth, hands, feet, or perineum, I would refer the child to the local specialist burns unit. Circumferential burns may require *escharotomy*.

REFERENCE

The Advanced Life Support Group 2001 Advanced paediatric life support — the practical approach. 3rd edn. BMJ Publishing Group

DROWNING

Q. Tell me about drowning and near-drowning.

Drownings and near-drowning accidents have an incidence of 1.5 per 100 000 children in the UK. The mortality is 0.7 per 100 000. Most accidents occur in inland fresh water, swimming pools and domestic baths and all are preventable.

Q. What do you know about the 'diving reflex'.

As soon as the face is submerged, breath-holding and bradycardia occurs. Continued breath-holding results in hypoxia, which leads to an increased heart rate and blood pressure, and acidosis. Eventually the person will attempt to breathe and fluid enters the mouth. The action of fluid touching the glottis results in severe laryngeal spasm and worsening hypoxia. Involuntary respiratory movements occur and fluid enters the lungs. (In 15% of drownings, the laryngeal spasm is so severe that fluid does not enter the lungs — 'dry drowning'.) Bradycardia, cardiac arrhythmia and cardiac arrest follow.

Q. Outline your management of a 10-year-old boy who is brought in to casualty after falling through the ice of a frozen lake while skating.

There are a number of important issues in the emergency management of near-drownings. I would want to take a detailed history from the ambulance staff who brought the child into hospital. In particular, I would want to know what resuscitation the child received at the scene, the length of time of submersion, and the time of the accident. The major problems that the child will encounter are hypoxia and hypothermia. I will deal with these in turn.

Hypoxia
My primary concern would be the child's airway, breathing and circulation. I would assess the airway, proceeding to intubation and ventilation with 100% oxygen if needed. I would assess the circulation, monitor the cardiac rhythm, and obtain intravenous access. If the child has a cardiac arrhythmia, I would follow the APLS guidelines for that arrhythmia. The child is likely to have swallowed water and I would pass a nasogastric tube to decompress the stomach.

Hypothermia
Given the history, I would expect this boy to be hypothermic. This can be advantageous. As soon as I have the child's ABC stabilised, I would insert a low-reading rectal thermometer to assess the core temperature. If the core temperature was >32°C I would use external warming with warm blankets

and radiant heaters. If the core temperature was <32°C I would give warm intravenous fluids at 37°C, ventilator gases at 42°C, and gastric/bladder lavage with normal saline at 42°C. I would also consider peritoneal dialysis with dialysate fluid at 42°C. ECMO is an alternative if available. I would not discontinue resuscitation until the child's core temperature had risen above 32°C.

REFERENCES

The Advanced Life Support Group 2001 Advanced paediatric life support – the practical approach. 3rd edn. BMJ Publishing Group
Sachdeva R C 1999. Near-drowning. Crit Care Clin 15: 281–296

CARDIAC ARRHYTHMIAS — EMERGENCY MANAGEMENT

Q. Tell us how you would manage asystole, pulseless electrical activity and ventricular fibrillation in a child.

These all demand immediate and appropriate action by adequately trained personnel. Familiarity with the location and operation of suitable equipment for efficient resuscitation is essential.

Although asystole and pulseless electrical activity (PEA) may have different aetiologies, their management is similar and I will discuss this followed by that for ventricular fibrillation. For each situation basic life support should precede management of the specific arrythymia.

Ventricular asystole / pulseless electrical activity (PEA)

For PEA, fluids should be given early (after the first dose of adrenaline). Diagnoses of exclusion are hypovolaemia, electrolyte disturbances ($\uparrow$ or $\downarrow$ potassium), hypothermia, tension pneumothorax, cardiac tamponade, pulmonary embolus and drug overdosage.

Other drugs may be used in the resuscitation process:

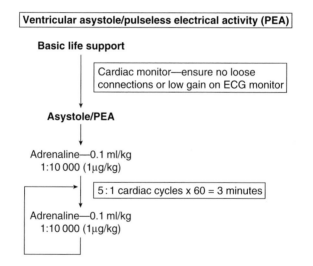

— NaHCO$_3$ — 1 mmol/kg = 1 ml/kg 8.4% sodium bicarbonate
— 10% dextrose — 5 ml/kg
— fluid boluses — 20 ml/kg 4.5% HAS / 0.9% normal saline
— atropine — 20 µg/kg. Minimum dose 100 µg, maximum dose 1000 µg

N.B. Sodium bicarbonate inactivates adrenaline. Flush the intravenous/intraosseus line between drug doses.

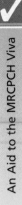
Ventricular fibrillation / tachycardia

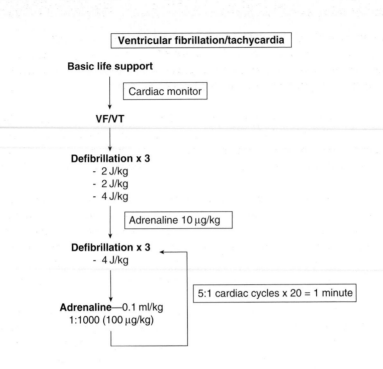

Other drugs considered in the resuscitation process:

— NaHCO₃, dextrose, fluid boluses as for asystole / PEA
— lignocaine — 1 mg/kg
— bretylium — 5 mg/kg

N.B. Modern defibrillators have the ability to pace externally. This is unlikely to be of use, except on PICU for children after cardiac surgery. In the newborn period complete heart block is usually diagnosed antenatally. Isoprenaline is the first-line treatment.

Tip

● You have got to know this like the back of your hand. No excuses, either in life or in the exam.

REFERENCE
The Advanced Life Support Group 2001 Advanced paediatric life support — the practical approach. 3rd edn. BMJ Publishing Group.

ELECTROLYTE PROBLEMS

Q. As the on-call paediatric registrar you are called by the surgical registrar to see a 2-year-old boy on a surgical ward who has been found to have a plasma sodium of 120 mmol/L. Tell me how you would manage this situation.

Hyponatraemia is defined as a plasma sodium below 130 mmol/L and is a relatively common problem in paediatric practice. In the situation you have described, I would expect that arming myself with the history, clinical findings, and some basic investigations would in most situations allow me to sort out the likely cause.

There are potentially grave complications of this metabolic derangement, most notably *cerebral impairment* and *convulsions*, and the likelihood of these will depend on the rapidity of the fall of the plasma sodium as well as the absolute level. It is important to unravel the underlying problem and direct treatment accordingly rather than simply to consider the plasma sodium alone. Indeed, inappropriate treatment may itself precipitate complications.

Whilst on the phone, I would establish from my surgical colleague whether the child is stable and not in need of immediate resuscitation. On arrival, I would briefly confirm that the sample is a genuine one and not one obtained 'upstream' from a drip-arm, which I have found to be a common explanation for this problem (especially in August!). I would also keep in mind the possibility of 'pseudo-hyponatraemia' in hyperlipidaemic or hyperproteinaemic states. This produces measured whole-plasma hyponatraemia with a normal concentration in plasma water and therefore at the cell surface.

I would then obtain a history from the surgical registrar, the parents if they were present, and from the case notes, paying particular attention to the reason for admission and what, if any, surgical procedures had been carried out. I would also enquire about the boy's general health, including perinatal history (?CAH), his general past medical and surgical history, and any recent problems such as diarrhoea or vomiting. Recent medication may be relevant in the case of prolonged steroid therapy or for various drugs that may cause inappropriate ADH secretion. I would also ask the surgical registrar to show me the treatment chart and any recent investigations. I would pay particular attention to the input/output chart and calculate the total fluid balance over the past few days taking note of what fluids had been used.

On examining the child, I would pay particular attention to the state of hydration, the pulse and blood pressure, and signs of peripheral oedema. I would also look for signs of chronic liver or renal disease and make my own subjective assessment of whether the child looked generally well or unwell.

I normally begin with a few basic investigations that may already be available, including the serum and urine electrolytes, blood glucose, and plasma and urine osmolality. In some situations, the blood gases may be important.

Based on my examination findings, I normally categorise the hypo-natraemia into one of three groups where there is:

1. A state of dehydration
2. Peripheral oedema
3. Clinically normal hydration

This simplifies the assessment and investigation of the possible causes of this boy's hyponatraemia which will in turn guide therapy.

The *dehydrated hyponatraemic* child suggests hypotonic dehydration with disproportionate loss of sodium over water. In this situation, the extracellular fluid is more hypotonic than intracellular fluid, which causes fluid shift into cells. This means that there is a serious risk of both *cerebral oedema* leading to convulsions, and a greater degree of shock per unit volume of fluid loss.

Careful questioning of the surgical registrar and the parents should exclude *gastroenteritis* or other causes of *vomiting* or *diarrhoea*. I would also consider other causes of gastrointestinal fluid loss such as *obstruction* or *fistulae* (? Crohn's disease). Losses from the skin due to severe *burns* will again be obvious. In all of these situations, the urinary sodium concentration will be low (below 20 mmol/L) as the body attempts to conserve total body sodium.

Other diagnoses that lead to *renal* loss of hypertonic fluid are:

— adrenal cortical hypofunction
— renal failure (diuretic phase)
— osmolar diuresis in DKA
— primary forms of renal tubular acidosis

A high plasma potassium (above 5.5 mmol/L) would favour the first three. If I found this picture together with a metabolic acidosis and low or low–normal plasma potassium, I would consider primary renal tubular acidosis as the likely cause.

Both renal failure and DKA should be readily identifiable from my basic investigations. *Adrenal cortical hypofunction* (due to congenital adrenal hyperplasia, prolonged steroid therapy, Addison's disease or fulminating infection) is an often forgotten and easily missed medical emergency that is particularly likely to manifest itself following the stress of surgery. I may have had clues to this diagnosis in the history (neonatal problems in CAH, steroid therapy) and examination (a child who looks unwell with unaccountable hypotension and weakness and, in Addison's disease, pigmentation). I would check the blood sugar to look for complicating *hypoglycaemia*. I would also be aware of the possibility of prominent GI symptoms being mistaken for gastroenteritis.

If I seriously suspected the diagnosis, especially in the face of the metabolic picture I have already described (or other features such as an elevated urea and hypochloraemic acidosis), I would perform a short *Synacthen test* (take blood for baseline plasma cortisol and then give 250 µg Synacthen (i.v. or i.m.), measuring plasma cortisol levels after 30 minutes and after 60 minutes). I would commence therapy as soon as I had taken the initial bloods and given the Synacthen if the clinical situation was sufficiently urgent. This would comprise i.v. normal saline fluid replacement (20 ml/kg), i.v. hydrocortisone sodium succinate 50 mg followed by 5 mg/kg per 24 hours in six divided doses, and correction of hypoglycaemia. Although hydrocortisone is essentially a glucocorticoid, it has sufficient mineralocorticoid activity to make it the drug of choice in the immediate management of both secondary and primary adrenal failure.

The results of the short Synacthen test would not be available immediately but would be interpretable even if I had to commence therapy. A normal 2–3-fold increase in plasma cortisol after Synacthen excludes the diagnosis of adrenal cortical hypofunction. I would bear in mind that hypotension with hyponatraemia, hyperkalaemia, and uraemia may be present in many acute clinical situations, as well as in an Addisonian crisis. However, it is still appropriate to treat blind if the diagnosis is suspected as there are few complications of this regimen and the consequences of delaying treatment of the condition may be grave.

Q. Tell me what your thoughts would be if you found this child to be oedematous.

Causes of hyponatraemia with oedema:

— hypoproteinaemic states such as nephrotic syndrome and liver disease (either chronic or fulminant)
— fluid-overload states such as injudicious fluid replacement (especially if dextrose solutions have been used), renal failure, and cardiac failure

Once again, a careful history and examination, inspection of the fluid-balance chart, and some basic blood and urine investigations should direct me towards the underlying cause. Daily weights (if they had been recorded) may also be very revealing.

Q. OK, tell me your thoughts if your examination found that the boy was neither dehydrated nor oedematous.

The most important cause of hyponatraemia with clinically normal hydration is the *syndrome of inappropriate ADH secretion (SIADH)*. Children seem particularly likely to show this metabolic reaction and common antecedent causes are respiratory illness, trauma (including surgical), and cerebral disease (such as trauma or infection). It may also be a complication of certain drugs such as opiates, carbamazepine or cytotoxics.

The diagnosis is based on the finding of hyponatraemia with a low plasma osmolality (below 270 mmol/kg) in the face of an inappropriately high urine osmolality or high urine sodium concentration (above 40 mmol/L). This will usually mean a urine:blood osmolality ratio >2 (i.e. a urine osmolality above 500 mmol/kg). However, the diagnosis should still be considered at levels short of this if the urine osmolality is considered to be inappropriately high with respect to the plasma value.

The complications are decreasing conscious level and convulsions that may be dangerously worsened by inappropriate fluid replacement if the condition is not recognised. The best management of SIADH is *fluid restriction* to 50% of normal which will result in slow restoration of plasma sodium and osmolality. In the acutely ill child, careful use of normal (which in any situation tends to normalise plasma osmolality) or even hypertonic saline, obeying strict regimens, may be justified. This must be done with extreme caution to avoid the cerebral complications or over-rapid correction of plasma osmolality. Paradoxically, diuretics such as furosemide(frusemide) are occasionally used to treat SIADH.

Other possible causes of this pattern are mild adrenocortical hypofunction or, again, injudicious fluid replacement. In both of these situations, the urine osmolality will not be inappropriately high.

Q. We have talked about abnormal sodium values — tell me how you would manage a child with a serum potassium that comes back from the laboratory as 8.5 mmol/L?

Not infrequently this is an erroneous result, arising from laboratory error or from haemolysis of the sample. For this reason, I would recheck the level, but in the meantime attach the child to a heart monitor and give nebulised salbutamol.

Q. What are you going to see on the monitor if the measurement is correct?

ECG findings in hyperkalaemia:

— tall T waves
— widening QRS complex
— broad, low amplitude P waves → disappears
— sine wave appearance

(ECG findings in *hypokalaemia* include: ↓ T-wave amplitude, U-wave appearance and ST-segment depression.)

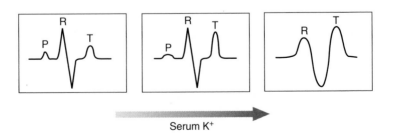

Serum K⁺

Q. OK, back to the question — how are you going to manage a serum potassium of 8.5 mmol/L, assuming it to be correct?

a) Stop all exogenous sources of potassium
b) ↑ pH of the acidotic patient by:
   — hyperventilation, if ventilated
   — $NaHCO_3$ — 1 mmol/kg or correct fully (weight (kg) × base excess × 0.3)
c) Nebulised salbutamol — continuous
d) 10% calcium gluconate: 0.5 ml/kg (0.1 mmol/kg) i.v. to stabilise the myocardium if arrythmias present
e) 20% dextrose: 2.5 ml/kg/hour i.v. centrally +/− insulin 0.05 units/kg/hour
f) Calcium resonium: 1 g/kg orally or rectally
g) Consider dialysis

Neonatology

3

HYPOGLYCAEMIA

Q. When would you consider it necessary to treat neonatal hypoglycaemia?

It is not clear what level of blood glucose is physiological for the newborn infant. The neonate has to adjust from a constant glucose supply in utero to an intermittent nutrient supply after birth. In the well term infant the surge of adrenaline at delivery causes the production of glucagon, cortisol and growth hormone, which allows gluconeogenesis and ketogenesis to proceed. In the first hour after birth, while these adaptations take place, the newborn term infant will have a lower blood glucose. This is physiological and probably does not require correction.

However, a low blood glucose after this initial period is potentially harmful. Traditionally, it has been thought that the newborn infant, particularly the premature infant, can tolerate a lower blood glucose than children and adults. This is because low plasma glucose concentrations are commonly demonstrated in newborn infants. There is, however, no evidence from the literature that the neonatal brain is less sensitive to hypoglycaemic injury than that of an older infant. More recent evidence suggests that recurrent episodes of hypoglycaemia (glucose levels <2.6 mmol/L), especially in small-for-gestational-age babies, are correlated with persistent neurodevelopmental delay and physical growth deficits up to 5 years of age.

One in ten normal term neonates cannot maintain plasma glucose concentrations above 1.7 mmol/L if their first feed is delayed beyond 3 to 6 hours of life. However, a single blood glucose level <2.6 mmol/L in a healthy term infant who is feeding well would not be of great concern, as a well baby can utilise alternative fuel supplies by the production of ketones. The *risk of hypoglycaemia* is greater for *preterm infants* who are unable to produce ketones and have little subcutaneous tissue to use in gluconeogenesis. Similarly, *small-for-gestational-age babies* have no substrate to use. Infants who have suffered *birth asphyxia* have also been found to have a reduced ketonic response and as these infants are often fluid restricted to prevent cerebral oedema, they are at increased risk of hypoglycaemia. *Infants of diabetic mothers* are prone to hypoglycaemia due to relative hyperinsulinism.

It is important to protect infants from hypoglycaemia by the introduction of early feeds. In the sicker infants intravenous glucose solutions should be started as soon after delivery as possible. Hypoglycaemia must then be treated vigorously should it occur. It has been shown that persistent moderate hypoglycaemia over a period of days is as potentially damaging as brief profound hypoglycaemia.

Further work is needed to clarify the definition of normoglycaemia for term and preterm infants down to the limit of viability. The long-term effects of persistent, intermittent, and brief profound episodes of hypoglycaemia on brain function and developemnt also warrant further study. Until the situation is clear, every attempt should be made to monitor accurately, and aggressively treat, low blood sugars in vulnerable neonates.

REFERENCES

Cornblath M, Hawdon J M, Williams A F et al 2000 Controversies regarding definition of neonatal hypoglycemia: suggested operational thresholds. Pediatrics 105: 1141–1145

Duvanel C B, Fawer C-L, Cotting J et al 1999 Long-term effects of neonatal hypoglycemia on brain growth and psychomotor development in small-for-gestational-age preterm infants. J Pediatr 134: 492–498

NECROTISING ENTEROCOLITIS

Q. Tell me what you know about NEC.

Necrotising enterocolitis is a relatively common disorder of unknown aetiology that primarily affects premature newborns, although around 7 to 13% of cases occur in full-term infants.

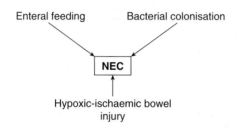

Hypoxic-ischaemic bowel injury with intestinal mucosal disruption in the presence of enteral feeding and bacterial colonisation may contribute to the development of NEC. Preterm and low-birth-weight infants have an increased susceptibility, presumably as a result of a compromised immune system. Numerous associations are described that further increase risk:

— congenital heart disease — ↓ cardiac output or R→L shunt, resulting in poor splanchnic perfusion
— umbilical vessel catheterisation
— polycythaemia → sludging of blood
— myelomeningocele — ? neurological disturbance to the intestine
— maternal cocaine use
— early and rapid enteral feeding, hyperosmolar feeds
— blood and exchange transfusions

At the molecular level, coagulation, necrosis, inflammation, and haemorrhage are seen. Nitric oxide is produced in large quantities by enterocytes in the intestinal wall. Extensive apoptosis is also demonstrated in the apical villi, suggesting that cytokine-induced NO production leads to apoptosis of the enterocyte and development of NEC.

Q. How could we try to prevent NEC occurring?

Because NEC primarily occurs in premature infants, prevention of preterm delivery would have a significant impact on its incidence. (This is a good viva subject in itself.) Measures to prevent preterm infants developing NEC are numerous:

— avoidance/minimisation of hypoglycaemia, hypoxia, systemic hypotension, exchange/blood transfusions

— careful nutritional management — judicious introduction of, and slow advancement of, oral feeding
— appropriate antibiotic therapy for specific infections

Other more contentious measures include:

— delivery by caesarean section for breech low birth weight infants. One study reported an incidence of NEC of 5.8% for vaginal delivery, compared with 0.6% for caesarian section
— high-frequency oscillation ventilation (HFOV) versus conventional ventilation for LBW infants. A multicentre study comparing modes of ventilation after surfactant administration in premature infants showed a significant decrease in suspected cases of NEC in the group given HFOV (6.2% vs. 19.7%)
— enteral or parenteral antibiotic prophylaxis. A Cochrane Review (1998) concluded that there was insufficient evidence to support this concept

Possible treatments for the future:

— continuous intraluminal perfusion of oxygenated perfluorocarbon for at-risk premature infants to ameliorate gut ischaemia
— prophylactic administration of platelet-activating-factor (PAF) blockers for at-risk infants. PAF-acetylhydrolase activity is seen in breast milk but not cow's milk, which may explain a higher incidence of NEC in formula-fed infants
— earlier detection of NEC, e.g. by gut nitric-oxide production, or by serum human-intestinal-fatty-acid-binding protein (hIFABP) — both elevated in the early phase of intestinal mucosal injury

Clusters or outbreaks of NEC appear to occur on NICUs. Whether this is coincidence, a reflection of the neonatal practice on that unit, or because of an unidentified infective agent associated with NEC development is difficult to interpret. However, strict infection-control measures to prevent cross-contamination are logical and easily incorporated into daily practice.

Key points

▲ 2–4% of infants admitted to NICUs develop NEC.

▲ The aetiology is unknown.

▲ Hypoxic-ischaemic bowel injury, bacterial colonisation of the gut, and the presence of intraluminal feeds may contribute to its development.

▲ The cessation of enteral feeds, commencement of i.v. fluids, oro-gastric drainage, parenteral antibiotics +/− surgery are the mainstay of treatment.

▲ Early detection of intestinal injury, e.g. NO production and serum hIFABP, may minimise overall damage.

Tip

● Extension of the discussion beyond NEC to incorporate the prevention of premature delivery, perfluorocarbon liquid ventilation, nitric oxide etc. is easily done. What examiner could resist something different from the subjects she has written down in front of her and will hear many times that day? In essence, you could almost choose the topics of discussion for the whole viva if you are persuasive and loquacious enough!

REFERENCES

Bury R G, Tudehope D 2000 Enteral antibiotics for preventing necrotising enterocolitis in low birthweight or preterm infants (Cochrane Review). In: The Cochrane Library, Issue 1. Update Software, Oxford

Craft A P, Finer N N, Barrington K J 2000 Vancomycin for prophylaxis against sepsis in preterm neonates (Cochrane Review). In: The Cochrane Library, Issue 1. Update Software, Oxford

Engum S A, Grosfeld J L 1998 Necrotizing enterocolitis. Curr Opin Pediatr 10: 123–130

BREASTFEEDING

Q. Tell me about breastfeeding.

Breastfeeding is the ideal method of infant nutrition and should be recommended to all new mothers. The advantages can be divided into those for the baby and those for the mother.

Advantages for the baby include:

1. An overall lower infant mortality rate.
2. Protection against infection by conveying IgA, lysozyme, lymphocytes, and macrophages — therefore transmitting both humoral and cellular immunity.
3. Breast milk is acidic and therefore promotes the growth of non-pathogenic, 'friendly' *lactobacillus* in the baby's bowel.
4. Breast milk contains *lactoferrin*, an iron-binding protein, which inhibits the growth of pathogenic *E.coli* and promotes the growth of *lactobacillus*.
5. In the first 2 or 3 days after birth the mother produces *colostrum* that is more yellow and watery than normal breast milk and is especially rich in IgA and contains some IgM. This is important in conferring early 'first-line' defences to the baby's GI tract. IgA protects the baby from both viral and bacterial infection.
6. The protein in breast milk is less likely to induce allergic reactions.
7. Babies born to atopic parents show a reduced tendency to eczema if breastfed.
8. Breast milk contains substances such as taurine and long- chain fatty acids, which are important for neurodevelopment (and may enhance IQ and visual acuity).
9. Breastfeeding is a natural way of promoting bonding between mother and baby.
10. Breastfeeding is more interesting for the baby as the maternal diet changes the taste!

Advantages for the mother include:

1. Breastfeeding is cheap, easy, convenient, and clean. It is supplied pre-prepared, pre-heated and sterile!
2. It is a 'total experience', stimulating all five senses and aiding the bonding process.
3. Suckling promotes uterine contraction, thereby reducing the risk of post-partum haemorrhage.
4. Full breastfeeding provides reasonable (but by no means guaranteed) contraception, due to the suppression of ovulation by prolactin.
5. Carcinoma of the breast is less common in women who have breastfed.

Q. What are the contraindications to breastfeeding?

There are few. *Maternal contraindications* include maternal HIV infection, maternal HbsAg-positive hepatitis B, maternal hepatitis C infection (only if co-infected with HIV), and certain legal and illegal drugs (see page 226).

Neonatal contraindications are certain inherited metabolic diseases such as PKU, galactosaemia, and mono- and disaccharide intolerance. Infants with anatomical abnormalities of the mouth, such as cleft palate, may be unable to breastfeed, but this is not an absolute contraindication.

Q. What are the differences between breast milk, cow's milk, and formula milk?

Breast milk contains about 70 kcal of energy per 100 ml compared with 66 kcal in cow's milk and 65 kcal in standard formula milks. There is considerably less protein in breast milk (1.0 g/dl compared to 1.8 g/dl for formula milk and 3.5 g/dl for cow's milk). Breast milk protein is composed largely of *whey*, which contains lactalbumin as well as lactoferrin and the immune proteins. Whey is more digestible than *caesin*, which is the major cow's-milk protein. Caesin is more likely to precipitate in the stomach as curd, which, though important in the regulation of stomach emptying, can lead to *curd obstruction*.

Breast milk contains a greater proportion of essential polyunsaturated fatty acids and cholesterol than cow's or formula milk. Bile-salt-stimulated lipase is present in breast milk only and is responsible for liberating fatty acids, which are important sources of energy for the baby.

Almost all the carbohydrate in the three types of milk is lactose, the amount in breast milk being considerably more than in cow's milk (7.5 g/dl compared with 5 g/dl) but about the same as in formula milk (7 g/dl). Lactose is easily metabolised to glucose and galactose (which is vital for normal myelin formation and brain development and is fermented by gut lactobacilli to produce an acid stool).

Breast milk has higher levels of vitamins A, C, and E than cow's milk, though less vitamin K, which may predispose to haemorrhagic disease of the newborn. The Department of Health recommends that vitamin drops are given to all breastfed babies.

I have already mentioned colostrum, which is produced in the first couple of days and is rather thin and watery and has a lower fat and carbohydrate content than milk. It is, however, rich in protein. Constituents also change during a feed, with milk at the end of a feed, hind milk, being richer in fat than foremilk. An infant who only takes the foremilk will not obtain maximum nutrition and may seem unsatisfied and fail to gain weight.

VENTILATION IN NEONATES

Q. Tell me about the various modes of ventilation you have experience of on the neonatal unit.

Essentially, standard mechanical ventilation can be divided into pressure-or volume-regulated control, or a combination of the two. From my experience, pressure-regulated ventilation is preferred in neonatal practice. In other words, the force or pressure required to push air/oxygen mix into the lungs is limited to reduce the risk of barotrauma. Tidal volume therefore depends on the pressures set and on the compliance of the lungs.

The standard mode for the preterm infant is *intermittent positive-pressure ventilation (IPPV)*. This delivers a tidal volume that is dependent on the pressure limits set by the operator i.e. it is pressure-regulated. Each breath is fully supported to the pressure set. Therefore, at a rate of 30 with pressures of 20/4, the ventilator will deliver a breath every 2 seconds to an inspiratory pressure of 20 cm water, keeping a closing pressure (or *PEEP*) of 4 cm water. This mode of ventilation is ideal for an infant with no spontaneous (or minimal) respiratory effort. *Synchronised IPPV* allows the ventilator to support any breaths taken by the baby to the pressures set provided the ventilator is sensitive enough to detect the patient's inspiratory effort. If a baby on SIPPV has a spontaneous respiratory rate of 60 and triggers the ventilator to support each of these breaths, altering the 'back-up' rate will have no effect unless it is increased above the baby's own respiratory rate. For this reason it is not an ideal mode for weaning from the ventilator.

A more suitable mode for weaning would be *synchronised intermittent mandatory ventilation (SIMV)*. This mode of ventilation will support the number of breaths that the ventilator has been set to give but will allow unsupported breaths in-between. Provided the baby breathes spontaneously at a rate faster than the rate set, all the ventilator breaths will be initiated by the baby. So, if a baby has a spontaneous respiratory rate of 60, without significant pauses, and the ventilator rate is 30, thirty breaths will be pressure supported and thirty will not be. Weaning can be initiated by reducing the number of breaths that are supported (by reducing the ventilator set-rate) so that the infant does more of the work of breathing himself.

'Patient-trigger ventilation' is a global term, simply describing the ventilator's ability to detect a signal which triggers it to deliver positive pressure during early inspiration. Signals can be derived from abdominal movement, thoracic impedance through electrocardiogram leads, or hot-wire anemometer wires detecting air flow. *Auto-cycling* is a potential problem in which flow sensors erroneously interpret secretions, water, hiccoughs, exogenous surfactant etc. as spontaneous respiratory effort and trigger the ventilator.

Modern ventilators offer further modes of ventilation such as pressure control, SIMV + pressure support, and pressure-regulated volume control (PRVC). I have limited experience of their use and I am unsure what additional benefit they confer over the more traditional modes of ventilation, particularly for neonates.

Q. What about high-frequency ventilation?

This form of ventilation uses supraphysiological ventilatory frequencies of 8–14 hertz (1 Hz = 60 b.p.m.). Low tidal volumes and low phasic pressure changes are generated within the lungs in an attempt to minimise volutrauma. This mode of ventilation can be used either as rescue in patients that are not adequately ventilated by methods described above or as initial therapy to try and avoid lung injury. Proponents suggest that higher ventilator mean airways pressure (MAP) should be used initially to avoid atelectasis and promote alveolar recruitment. Once optimal lung volume is achieved, functional residual capacity is maintained and the large swings in airway pressure associated with inflation and deflation seen with conventional ventilation are avoided. Infant studies have, however, not shown the significant benefit from HFOV seen with animal studies, when compared with conventional ventilation.

Q. Do you know about any other forms of ventilation?

Although I have very little experience (or none) of *negative extrathoracic pressure* (NEP) ventilation, I know that some units in the UK have studied its use in premature infants. Although initial results appeared promising, a secondary analysis of the data showed that continuous NEP was associated with increased mortality, cranial ultrasound abnormalities, and pneumothoraces.

Similarly, my experience of *extracorporeal membranous oxygenation* (ECMO) is limited to an occasional sick neonate being transferred to an ECMO centre because of failure of conventional ventilatory methods. ECMO is essentially a modified technique of cardiac bypass that *allows prolonged respiratory support* while minimising the barotrauma caused by standard mechanical ventilation. Blood is drained from an artery or vein, passes through a membrane oxygenator, and is then re-warmed and infused back into the carotid artery. The UK Collaborative ECMO Trial Group reported a mortality rate of 30% for neonates randomised to ECMO compared with 59% in those given conventional ventilation. Contraindications to its use include a body weight less than 2 kg, gestational age less than 35 weeks, significant intraventricular haemorrhage, irreversible lung disease, age greater than 10 days, and significant congenital anomaly. Its major complication is bleeding.

I have read a little about liquid ventilation, although I am not aware of any centres in the UK using this technique, except in the laboratory. Perfluorocarbons are inert, non-toxic, colourless and odourless liquids with low surface tension and high oxygen and carbon dioxide affinity. The technique involves filling the lungs to functional residual capacity and then applying conventional gas ventilation via the endotracheal tube. Elimination of the liquid occurs by evaporation. I look forward to seeing the results of randomised controlled studies using this form of ventilation!

Tips

- Oxgen index = $\dfrac{\text{mean airway pressure} \times \text{Fio}_2 \times 100}{\text{PaO}_2}$

- ECMO should be considered for a neonate with an oxygen index over 35–40.

REFERENCES

Biarent D 1999 New tools in ventilatory support: high- frequency ventilation, nitric oxide, tracheal gas insufflation, non-invasive ventilation. Pediatr Pulmonol 18: 178–181

McGettigan M C, Adolph V R, Ginsberg H G et al 1998 New ways to ventilate newborns in acute respiratory failure. Pediatr Clin N Am 45: 475–509

UK Collaborative ECMO Trial Group 1996 UK collaborative randomised trial of neonatal extracorporeal membrane oxygenation. Lancet 348: 75–82

Weis C M, Fox W W 1999 Current status of liquid ventilation. Curr Opin Pediatr 11: 126–132

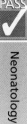
MILKS FOR NEONATES

Q. Does it matter which milk we feed infants?

Current Department of Health guidelines advise that newborn infants should be exclusively breastfed for at least the first 4 months of life, with solid feeds being introduced after this point. The benefits of breastfeeding for both mother and infant are numerous (see page 76). For the infant, these benefits include:

— a reduction in the incidence of gastroenteritis, respiratory illnesses, and atopy
— improved visual acuity — at least, possibly, in the short term
— increased intelligence quotient — contentious!

The benefits breast milk conveys to the infant are related to its content. Immunoglobulin A, lysozyme, lymphocytes and macrophages, all present in breast milk, contribute to this enhanced protection against infection. Lactoferrin is also present and inhibits colonisation of the gut with pathogenic *Escherichia coli* as well as promoting the growth of lactobacilli within the gut. Breast milk contains small amounts of long-chain polyunsaturated fatty acids (LCPUFA) that are thought to promote visual acuity and improve IQ.

Q. Tell me about LCPUFAs

The essential fatty acids, linoleic acid and α-linolenic acid can be desaturated and elongated by specific enzymes to produce LCPUFAs — primarily arachidonic and docosahexanoic acids. Arachidonic acid is the precursor of the eicosanoids, leukotrienes, thromboxanes, and prostaglandin. Arachidonic acid and docosahexanoic acid are the major components of phospholipids, which are found in abundance in cellular membranes. Breast milk contains small amounts of these LCPUFAs but unsupplemented formula milks do not and it has been shown that visual acuity at 4 months of age is better in breastfed infants than in formula-fed infants. This is particularly apparent in preterm infants in whom the metabolic pathways for elongation and desaturation of fatty acids are immature. Similarly, children given mother's milk in early infancy have demonstrated higher IQs than children who have never received breast milk.

Q. What, then, should we be feeding preterm infants with?

Standard milk formulae and non-fortified breast milk do not fully meet the nutritional needs of the premature infant. If available, fortified human breast milk should therefore be used. If breast milk is unavailable, a preterm formula should be given, which provides more protein, fat, calcium, phosphate, vitamins, and trace elements than term milk formulae. There is considerable

debate as to whether or not preterm formulae should be supplemented with LCPUFAs. Proponents suggest that nutritional intervention during sensitive periods in early life can have a major impact in later life (the 'Barker hypothesis' — see page 280); detractors claim that short-term alteration in the phospholipid content of the brain and retina have little if any impact on long-term function. There is therefore a need for long-term prospective nutrition-intervention studies to examine these differences of opinion.

Q. What about glutamine supplementation for preterm infants?

This again is a contentious issue and requires prospective randomised controlled trials to determine whether supplementation enhances gut integrity and reduces sepsis rates in the newborn period. Glutamine is the commonest amino acid found in plasma and muscle, and is used as the primary energy source by rapidly proliferating cells such as enterocytes and lymphocytes. By enhancing gut mucosal integrity, glutamine supplementation in preterm infants may expedite tolerance of enteral feeds. Improved lymphocyte function may also reduce the incidence of sepsis. A number of trials in preterm infants suggest a benefit but a recent Cochrane Review failed to conclude, from the evidence to date, that glutamine supplementation is advantageous.

Tip

● The subject of breastfeeding commonly comes up in the viva. Questions may include: the content of breast milk compared with formula milk and cow's milk; the incidence of breastfeeding and measures to improve breastfeeding rates (Our Healthier Nation); and the contraindications to breastfeeding. It is a bit of a 'touchy-feely' subject and worth knowing in detail!

REFERENCES

Kurlak L O, Stephenson T J 1999 Plausible explanations for effects of long-chain polyunsaturated fatty acids (LCPUFA) on neonates. Arch Dis Child Fet Neonat Edn 80: F148–F154

Tubman T R J, Thompson S W. Glutamine supplementation for preventing morbidity in preterm infants (Cochrane Review). In: The Cochrane Library, 2, 2001. Update Software, Oxford

Wilson A C, Forsyth J S, Greene S A et al 1998 Relation of infant diet to childhood health: seven-year follow-up of cohort of children in Dundee infant feeding study. Br Med J 316: 21–25

BONE DISEASE OF PREMATURITY

Q. What can you tell us about the metabolic bone disease of prematurity?

Most calcium and phosphorus accretion occurs in fetal bones during the last trimester of pregnancy, when the minerals are actively transported across the placenta. This means that phosphate and calcium stores are low in infants born before term and explains why we are seeing an increased incidence of metabolic bone disease, now that infants of less than 30 weeks gestation have improved survival rates. Maternal pre-eclampsia increases the risk of metabolic bone disease, presumably as a result of reduced transfer of phosphate and calcium across the unhealthy placenta.

Metabolic bone disease of infancy develops due to *low phosphate intake*, which causes poor deposition of minerals in cartilage and bone. It is therefore more common in those infants fed on breast milk, because the concentration of phosphate in breast milk is lower than that in formula milk. It is also more common in those infants requiring a period of *total parenteral nutrition*, because it is difficult to put adequate concentrations of calcium and phosphate into solution without causing precipitation of salts. Most infants have adequate production of active vitamin D from the kidney, so absorption of calcium and phosphate from the intestine is not usually a problem.

Metabolic bone disease can be recognised by high levels of alkaline phosphatase in the absence of liver disease. Osteopenia of the metaphyseal plate may be seen on X-rays of the wrist or knee, but it is usually quite severe before it is recognised. Measurement of bone density would identify osteopenia earlier, but is not practical in these infants as a routine. In severe cases, there will be fraying and cupping of the metaphysis and fractures may be identified (particularly of the ribs). It is unusual to be able to detect these findings clinically, although an infant may experience increasing respiratory distress as a result of osteopenia of the ribs.

Q. How would you treat an infant with metabolic bone disease?

Ideally, I would like to prevent it. I would give oral phosphate supplements to preterm infants who are on breast milk. Although metabolism of vitamin D should be normal, vitamin D is sometimes given to preterm or unwell infants to supplement intake. If calcium levels were low in the presence of a high alkaline phosphatase, I would also give calcium supplements. However, calcium should *always* be accompanied by phosphate to avoid deposition of excess calcium in the kidneys, causing nephrocalcinosis.

Key points

▲ Preterm infants have acquired less maternal calcium and phosphate than term infants.

▲ Low phosphate intake causes metabolic bone disease.

▲ Alkaline phosphatase levels are an indicator of bone turnover.

POLYCYTHAEMIA

Q. What do you know about polycythaemia in neonates?

Polycythaemia is due to a raised red blood cell volume, which may be due to *red cell transfusion* or occurred as a response to *intrauterine hypoxia*. Red cell transfusion may be from twin to twin, from the placenta, or due to delayed clamping of the umbilical cord. Intrauterine hypoxia occurs with placental insufficiency, which may be due to maternal hypertension, smoking, or post-maturity. The infant may be small-for-dates. Other infants at risk of polycythaemia are infants of diabetic mothers and infants with trisomy 21.

The infant may present with plethora, lethargy, poor feeding, hypotonia, irritability and jittery movements. The plethora may get worse in the first 24 hours as the plasma volume drops.

Polycythaemia is confirmed on blood sampling. A capillary sample will have a higher haematocrit than a peripheral venous sample. A sample of arterial or central venous blood should be used when possible, as testing of peripheral blood will cause over-diagnosis of polycythaemia. Ideally, the specimen should be measured by centrifugation in the neonatal unit, as laboratory values are based on derived numbers of red cells and tend to show a lower packed cell volume than a centrifuged specimen. A haematocrit of more than 0.65 is considered to be indicative of polycythaemia. However, some infants are symptomatic with a haematocrit of 0.6.

Polycythaemic infants are at risk of *intravascular thromboses*, which may affect the cerebral vessels, increasing the risk of seizures as well as significant neurodevelopmental disability. They may also develop renal vein thromboses and are at a higher risk of necrotising enterocolitis. Polycythaemic infants also have a tendency to hypoglycaemia and hypocalcaemia, thrombocytopenia, and jaundice.

Symptomatic infants need treatment. Initially, the aim is to maintain hydration, but if there is significant polycythaemia, *partial exchange transfusion* may be necessary. I tend to use partial exchange if the haematocrit is above 0.65 in a symptomatic infant, or above 0.7 in an asymptomatic infant. I use fresh frozen plasma or human albumin solution for the exchange and use a peripheral arterial and venous line where possible, as there is an increased risk of thrombosis after cannulating the umbilical vessels.

INTRAVENTRICULAR HAEMORRHAGE

Q. How would you classify intraventricular haemorrhage in the preterm infant?

Intraventricular haemorrhage (IVH) can be classified according to the location and extent of the haemorrhage seen on cranial ultrasound. In preterm infants the bleeding originates in the highly vascular *germinal matrix*. The germinal matrix shrinks as the infant approaches term, and in term infants the source of IVH is usually the *choroid plexus*.

The haemorrhage may be confined to the germinal matrix or extend into the ventricular system. The extent of the spread into the ventricles and the presence of dilatation of the ventricles should be recorded.

Intraventricular haemorrhage can be classified in four grades:

Grade I — germinal matrix or subependymal haemorrhage
Grade II — intraventricular haemorrhage with no ventricular distension
Grade III — intraventricular haemorrhage with ventricular distension
Grade IV — periventricular haemorrhage

It used to be thought that grade IV haemorrhage had extended through the ventricular wall into the parenchyma, but it is now accepted that it is due either to venous infarction or to haemorrhage into a pre-existing periventricular infarct, which might have been caused by an hypoxic event.

Q. What are the causes of intraventricular haemorrhage?

Sudden *surges in blood pressure* may cause IVH, so prevention should be aimed at reducing stressors that might cause a sudden change in blood pressure. Regular endotracheal suction and unpleasant stimuli should be avoided where possible and the infant should be sedated so that invasive procedures are less distressing. Early *hypotension* is also thought to increase the chances of IVH, as ischaemia will increase the fragility of blood vessels.

Other risk factors for IVH include an *increase in partial pressure of carbon dioxide* and *hypoxia*, which cause vasodilatation of cerebral blood vessels. For this reason, careful monitoring of ventilation in order to avoid dramatic changes in gas exchange is important.

Q. How would you recognise intraventricular haemorrhage clinically?

It may not be possible to detect IVH clinically, although there may be an episode of clinical deterioration associated with metabolic acidosis and anaemia in some cases. The anterior fontanelle may be found to be bulging in the presence of a large bleed. More usually, the presence of IVH is detected on routine cranial ultrasound. This is usually performed a few days after birth, as haemorrhage is most common at this time. I would arrange a more urgent scan if there were any neurological signs, such as seizures, or clinical suspicion of intracranial haemorrhage. If there was an IVH present, I would arrange a second scan towards the end of the first week in order to ascertain the maximum degree of extension. If the IVH extended beyond the germinal matrix, scans should be performed at two-weekly intervals in order to detect post-haemorrhagic hydrocephalus or periventricular haemorrhagic infarction.

Q. What is the mechanism for hydrocephalus in this situation?

Hydrocephalus occurs as a result of impaired reabsorption of cerebrospinal fluid, secondary to blockage of the arachnoid villi by particulate matter or obstruction of the aqueduct of Sylvius by clot. There is a delay between the development of ventricular dilatation and the appearance of clinical signs of hydrocephalus, so it is important to perform serial ultrasound scans to measure the ventricular size.

Q. What treatment will be required?

In many cases ventriculomegaly will resolve with time, so there is a case for watchful waiting. However, if there is progressive dilatation, a surgical procedure is necessary. In a minority of cases, serial lumbar punctures may be useful, but most infants require a ventriculostomy or insertion of a ventriculoperitoneal shunt. A recent trial looked at the use of acetazolamide in the treatment of post-haemorrhagic hydrocephalus, but my understanding is that no benefit was demonstrated.

JAUNDICE

Q. Outline your management of jaundice in newborn babies.

Jaundice can be divided into physiological jaundice, jaundice developing in the first 24 hours, jaundice developing in the first week, and prolonged jaundice.
I will go through these in order:

Physiological jaundice
Seen in 50% of term babies and 80% of premature infants, this is the result of rapid breakdown of fetal haemoglobin and the immaturity of liver conjugating enzymes. An elevated unconjugated serum bilirubin is seen and most cases require no further investigation.

Jaundice in the first 24 hours
Jaundice occurring at this stage is usually due to haemolysis.

a) Aetiology:
   — physiological
   — ABO or rhesus incompatibility
   — red cell membrane abnormalities (spherocytosis, elliptocytosis)
   — red cell enzyme defects (G6PD, pyruvate kinase)
   — congenital infection
b) Investigations:
   — FBC + film
   — bilirubin
   — blood group
   — Coombs' test
   — TORCH screen
c) Treatment:
Dependent on the cause. I would be guided by bilirubin charts but most will require phototherapy and some will need exchange transfusion.

Jaundice in the first week

a) Aetiology:
   — physiological
   — sepsis
   — hypothyroidism
b) Investigations:
   — Full septic work up including LP and urine culture
   — TFT
   — FBC + film
   — bilirubin
   — blood group
   — Coombs' test

c) Treatment:
— i.v. antibiotics for sepsis
— phototherapy/exchange transfusion
— thyroxine for hypothyroidism

Prolonged Jaundice (> 14 days)

a) Aetiology:
— physiological (breast milk) jaundice
— biliary atresia
— cystic fibrosis
— α_1-antitrypsin deficiency
— galactosaemia
— anatomical abnormalities
b) Investigations:
— FBC
— split bilirubin
— LFTs
— urine reducing substances, bilirubin
— α_1-antitrypsin phenotype
— sweat test

Any baby that is still jaundiced at 14 days requires immediate investigation to exclude extrahepatic biliary atresia (EHBA). The 1993 'Yellow Alert' National Awareness Campaign was launched to increase public awareness and hopefully promote early diagnosis and referral for surgery.

Q. Tell me about the operative treatment of biliary atresia.

The operation of choice in extrahepatic biliary atresia is a *Kasai's hepato-portoenterostomy*: a Roux-en-Y of jejunum is brought up, closed at its end and anastomosed to the porta hepatis; the proximal divided jejunum is anastomosed to the side of the Roux loop to keep the bowel contents away from the porta hepatis. The prognosis for EHBA is related to age at surgery, with 90% of those under 2 months achieving drainage of bile. Those presenting over 3 months of age are unlikely to obtain successful drainage. *Complications* of the procedure include ascending bacterial cholangitis and portal hypertension. Biliary atresia is the commonest single indication for liver transplantation in children.

REFERENCE
Middlesworth W et al 1997 Biliary atresia. Curr Opin Pediatr 9: 265–269

ANTENATAL SCREENING

Q. What antenatal screening takes place in the UK?

Ideally, all prospective parents planning to have a family should attend their GP for general advice prior to conception. The GP can advise regarding smoking; alcohol consumption; stopping contraception; diet; maintenance of good glycaemic control for patients with diabetes; avoidance of potentially teratogenic drugs; and use of vitamin and folate supplementation.

Screening starts when a prospective mother first attends the GP to confirm the pregnancy (usually when the second period has been missed). Every woman should have blood taken for haemoglobin (screening for anaemia), blood group (to identify rhesus-negative women), rubella status, syphilis serology and hepatitis B serology. Hepatitis C and HIV serology should be performed in high-risk pregnancies. In addition to a full history and examination, an assessment of risk for the pregnancy should be made. High-risk pregnancies — poor obstetric history, older mothers, and complex medical problems — should be referred early to the obstetrician. The standard procedure for 'normal risk' pregnancies is *shared care* between the GP and hospital with antenatal visits every 6–8 weeks until 28 weeks, then fortnightly until 36 weeks, and thereafter weekly until delivery. At all visits, mothers should be weighed, their blood pressure measured (to identify pregnancy-induced hypertension at an early stage), their urine dipsticked for protein and glucose (to exclude UTI, gestational diabetes), the fundal height palpated and fetal heart auscultated.

In many centres pregnant women have a *booking ultrasound scan* of the fetus and placenta. Ideally, this should be performed before 15 weeks gestation. This scan will accurately establish gestational age (<13 weeks—crown–rump length; >13 weeks — biparietal diameter and/or head circumference), viability and fetal number. The *'anomaly scan'* is performed in many centres at 20 weeks gestation. This will assess the detailed anatomy of the baby and assess the position and condition of the placenta. The volume of amniotic fluid volume is also assessed. Major structural abnormalities such as spina bifida, anencephaly, major congenital heart disease and kidney abnormalities are easily diagnosed. With increasingly refined ultrasound technology, small anatomical defects can now be identified, which may or may not be productive. On the one hand, forewarned is forearmed; but on the other, knowledge may create anxiety, often out of proportion to the degree of abnormality.

Q. I'll stop you there. What specific tests are used in screening for Down's syndrome?

There have been numerous advances in the antenatal screening for Down's syndrome. The original *'triple test'* is a blood test taken between 15 and 22 weeks of pregnancy, which measures α-fetoprotein (AFP), unconjugated oestriol (uE$_3$) and human chorionic gonadotrophin (hCG). The results, together with maternal age and assessment of gestational age by ultrasound, give a detection rate (for a 5% false-positive rate) of 69%. This test has recently been improved by additionally measuring serum inhibin-A, increasing the detection rate to 76% (the *quadruple test*).

Considerable research has been centred on finding more specific, earlier markers of Down's syndrome. It has been shown that the condition is associated with increased serum free β-hCG and decreased pregnancy-associated plasma protein-A (PAPP-A). When combined with maternal age, an increased *fetal nuchal translucency* on ultrasound at 10–14 weeks gestation gives a detection rate of 62%.

Recently, a combination of first- and second-trimester tests has been introduced (the *integrated test*). This involves measuring serum PAPP-A and nuchal translucency by ultrasound in the first trimester and serum AFP, uE$_3$, hCG and inhibin-A in the second trimester. This combination of investigations has a detection rate of 85% with a false-positive rate of 0.9%.

From these investigations a *risk score* can be calculated. Those with a score of 1 in 250 or less are considered screening-positive and are offered a diagnostic test either by amniocentesis or by chorionic villus sampling (CVS). Both of these invasive procedures, however, carry a risk of miscarriage (amniocentesis — 1%; CVS — 1.5%).

Q. Are you aware of any recent developments in this field?

A great deal of research interest has been centred on identifying markers of Down's syndrome in maternal urine. To date the results are inconclusive, although increased urinary β-core-fragment of hCG, free β-hCG and hyperglycosylated hCG are seen in the second trimester. There are no clinically useful urinary markers in the first trimester.

Fetal DNA can be extracted from maternal blood in pregnancy. In principle, it is easy to diagnose Down's syndrome from this but extraction of the DNA is technically difficult and expensive.

REFERENCES
Cuckle H 2000 Biochemical screening for Down's syndrome. Eur J Obstet Gynaecol Reprod Biol 92: 97–101
Royal College of Obstetricians and Gynaecologists 2000 Routine ultrasound screening in pregnancy. Protocol, standards and training. RCOG, London
Wald N J et al 1999 Integrated screening for Down's syndrome based on tests performed during the first and second trimester. N Engl J Med 341: 461–467

INBORN ERRORS OF METABOLISM

Q. What might lead you to consider an inborn error of metabolism in an infant?

The features of inborn errors of metabolism (IEM) are often non-specific and it is important to have a low threshold of suspicion. Early recognition of metabolic disorders may allow effective treatment for some conditions, preventing permanent hepatic, renal, or cerebral damage.

Inborn errors of metabolism are less common than sepsis in the newborn and many of the presenting features, such as lethargy, poor feeding and hypotonia, are similar. Most infants will therefore quite rightly be treated for sepsis initially. Clues to the diagnosis include a family history of neonatal death or consanguinity (many of the disorders are autosomal recessive). Improvement on intravenous fluids with further deterioration once enteral feeds are restarted is also suggestive. Other clinical features include neurological problems, such as drowsiness and convulsions, vomiting, jaundice, and hepatomegaly. The infant may have persistent hypoglycaemia or an unusual odour of the urine.

It can be difficult to pinpoint the diagnosis clinically, so investigations should be broad initially. I check plasma glucose, sodium, potassium, calcium, bicarbonate, urea, creatinine, and liver function tests in the first instance. I would also check a urine specimen for reducing substances if jaundice and hypoglycaemia were a feature, as this may point towards a diagnosis of galactosaemia. However, reducing substances may be negative in a vomiting infant and I would check the enzyme galactose-1-phosphate uridyltranferase if the diagnosis was likely.

I would consider checking plasma ammonia, particularly if the infant had altered consciousness. This will help diagnose urea cycle disorders, which may present with hypoglycaemia, liver impairment and neurological symptoms. Ammonia may also be mildly raised in any sick infant, however, so results must be interpreted with caution. Plasma lactate may be useful as it is raised in infants with defects of the pyruvate dehydrogenase complex, although it is also high in many children with poor peripheral perfusion. I would collect plasma and urine for analysis by amino acid chromatography and send urine for organic acid analysis and ketones.

Q. Can you give us an example of an amino acid disorder?

The most common disorder of amino acid metabolism is maple syrup urine disease, which might present with poor feeding, vomiting, drowsiness and seizures, with an associated metabolic acidosis. It may be possible to detect a sweet odour from the infant. There is a defect in breakdown of the three branched-chain amino acids, leucine, valine, and isoleucine, leading to their accumulation in all body compartments. It may be necessary to start peritoneal dialysis in order to reduce the levels of plasma amino acids.

If the condition is diagnosed promptly it may be possible to prevent brain damage by dietary manipulation. The infant requires protein restriction and 'special' formula milk, manufactured to replace amino acids, but containing no branched-chain amino acids. Since the branched-chain amino acids are essential, regulated amounts of natural protein would be allowed. It is possible to monitor blood spot levels of valine, leucine and isoleucine regularly in order to make any necessary dietary adjustments.

Q. Fine. Now give us an example of an inborn error of metabolism that would be diagnosed from organic acid analysis in the neonatal period.

Disturbances of fatty acid metabolism, such as long-chain acyl CoA dehydrogenase deficiency, may cause abnormalities on organic acid analysis, with an increase in dicarboxylic acids. These conditions rarely present in the newborn period, but may become apparent in the first few months of life. Beta-oxidation of fatty acids is essential for energy production in the stressed or starved infant, so if an infant with one of these conditions is not taking feeds, they develop hypoglycaemia and lethargy. The infant improves on intravenous dextrose fluids, since an alternative energy source is being provided. A urine specimen will show no ketones in the presence of hypoglycaemia, which should give a clue to the diagnosis before the organic acid analysis is available. Treatment relies on adequate provision of carbohydrate, particularly at times of stress, with supplementary carnitine, which is required for transport of fatty acids into mitochondria.

Tip

● Remember — only offer diagnoses that you are confident about. The examiners will not always pick you up on specific topics, for example urea cycle defects in the above question, but it is not a risk worth taking!

ETHICAL DILEMMAS ON THE NEONATAL UNIT

Q. What are your views on the ethics of neonatal medicine?

Due to advances in technology, no other medical speciality has more ethical dilemmas than neonatology. Every day the neonatologist is faced with the decision, 'Shall I or shall I not treat?' No two situations are the same and no two neonatologists would always agree in the same situation. Very often the decision to continue or not (or indeed start) is in the hands of the most junior doctor who is present on the baby unit 24 hours a day. The decision made by the attending doctor must be made in the patient's best interest.

In 1997, the Royal College of Paediatrics and Child Health published a report on the withholding and withdrawing of life-saving treatment. In this report there are five situations where withdrawal or withholding of treatment might be considered:

1. *The brain-dead child* — brainstem-death tests must be performed by two medical practitioners.
2. *The permanent vegetative state.*
3. *The 'no-purpose' situation.*
4. *The 'no-chance' situation* — where treatment is merely delaying death.
5. *The 'unbearable' situation* — where parents and/or the child feel that further treatment is more than can be borne.

Specific to neonatal practice, clinical situations where treatment may not be started, may be discontinued, or may be limited include:

— non-resuscitation of a baby at birth with a congenital abnormality that is incompatible with life, e.g. anencephaly
— non-resuscitation of a baby born of <23 weeks gestation. The parents must accept that it is the neonatologist's opinion that if the baby survives the risks of severe neurological impairment are extremely high and that many weeks of intensive care cannot be justified
— withdrawal of artificial ventilation in a baby who has suffered birth asphyxia where there is evidence of profound brain damage on investigation (ultrasound scan, CT, MRI, EEG)

Q. What are the views of the RCPCH on euthanasia?

The RCPCH is strongly against euthanasia. Administering a drug with the intention of hastening death is unlawful. However, administering a drug to relieve suffering, which may as a side-effect hasten death, is lawful. If muscle-paralysing drugs were being used in the child *prior* to the decision to withdraw care then they do not need to be discontinued. However, they should not be started prior to withdrawal of care if they were not previously clinically indicated.

REFERENCE

The Royal College of Paediatrics and Child Health 1997 Withholding or withdrawing life-saving treatment in children. RCPCH, London

Neonatology

NEONATAL METABOLIC ACIDOSIS

Q. What would you consider when a preterm infant develops metabolic acidosis?

Metabolic acidosis is a common finding in the premature infant. Firstly, I would check how the sample had been obtained. If it was taken by heel prick from a newborn infant, for example, the sample might be affected by poor perfusion in the extremities. Ideally, I would obtain an arterial blood sample to confirm a low bicarbonate level and negative base excess. The pH is likely to be low, unless the infant is tachypnoeic or over-ventilated.

The differential diagnosis includes *infection, hypoxia* and *dehydration*. All of these cause poor peripheral perfusion and are common in the susceptible preterm infant. I would assess the infant for signs of hypovolaemia, such as tachycardia, hypotension, and reduced capillary return. I would give a bolus of 10 ml/kg 0.9% saline to see if the perfusion improved, with a further dose if the clinical response was inadequate. I would do a septic screen and start broad-spectrum antibiotics, such as penicillin and gentamicin, if there were any risk factors for sepsis. If the acidosis persisted, I might consider slow intravenous infusion of 4.2% sodium bicarbonate solution. However, sodium bicarbonate has a high osmolality and causes changes in intracellular osmolality and, potentially, cerebral oedema, so should be avoided if possible. THAM is an alternative alkaline solution and has a lower sodium content. It can cause apnoea and should not be used unless the infant is being ventilated.

Hypovolaemia secondary to *haemorrhage,* for example intraventricular haemorrhage, may cause acidosis and I would perform a cranial ultrasound in an infant with unexplained metabolic acidosis. If this confirms intraventricular haemorrhage, I would use blood as volume replacement, as this will correct the acidosis more reliably.

Poor circulation secondary to severe *congenital heart defects,* such as hypoplastic heart syndrome, will cause metabolic acidosis and might be difficult to detect on clinical examination. A chest X-ray would show cardiomegaly and plethoric lung fields, and the ECG would show signs of right ventricular hypertrophy and right axis deviation.

Persistent metabolic acidosis may be the result of *total parenteral nutrition* (TPN) in the preterm infant. The solution is often quite acidic and may vary on a daily basis. If this is thought to be the cause, it may be necessary to run a separate infusion of low-dose sodium bicarbonate while TPN continues.

Other causes of metabolic acidosis include *renal impairment*, when generation of bicarbonate is reduced, and metabolic disorders. Further investigations would be justified if the metabolic acidosis remained unexplained.

HYPOXIC ISCHAEMIC ENCEPHALOPATHY

Q. Tell me about hypoxic ischaemic encephalopathy.

Hypoxic ischaemic encephalopathy (HIE) is a neurological syndrome caused by asphyxial injury to the perinatal brain. Its incidence is around 6 per 1000 live term births. Very simply, hypoxia (reduced oxygen content of the blood) and/or ischaemia (reduced blood perfusion in the tissues), from whatever cause, result in ATP depletion, cessation of normal cellular function, and neuronal cell death. Depending on the duration and severity of asphyxia and the subsequent resuscitation process, three clinical grades of severity are described:

Grade 1 (mild) — poor suck, brisk reflexes, mild hypotonia, hyperalertness, uninhibited Moro reflex

Grade 2 (moderate) — lethargy, absent suck, hypotonia, decreased spontaneous movements, convulsions very common

Grade 3 (severe) — stupor/coma, flaccid tone, prolonged fits, absent suck and Moro reflexes, bulbar and autonomic dysfunction

The diagnosis is essentially clinical although there are a number of useful investigations which aid in assessment of severity and prognosis: EEG can show background and epileptic activity and the presence or absence of burst suppression; Doppler ultrasound can assess cranial blood flow; serial cranial ultrasonography and computerised tomography can demonstrate the development of selective neuronal necrosis; and finally, MRI can give detailed information about the distribution and extent of hypoxic injury, although long-term prognosis in survivors is still difficult to predict from this.

Q. You mentioned that ischaemia and/or hypoxia are the cause of HIE. Can you give more detail than this at the cellular level?

Normally, ATP production for cellular processes within the brain is from aerobic glucose metabolism. If oxygen is unavailable glucose is metabolised anaerobically but produces only about 6% of the ATP produced aerobically. Lactate and pyruvate accumulate and a metabolic acidosis develops. If the asphyxial injury continues, ATP rapidly becomes depleted. Cellular processes, such as the ATP-dependent sodium–potassium pump, fail with influx of sodium and calcium into the cell. Glutamate is released during an hypoxic-ischaemic injury. This excitatory neurotransmitter opens the NMDA channel on the surface of brain cells, which also allows calcium influx. Brain ischaemia and reperfusion induces an inflammatory response with release of cytokines (IL-1 and IL-6), platelet-activating factor and other factors. All these processes result in oxygen free-radical production that uncouples oxidative phosphorylation within the mitochondria, and cell death ensues.

97

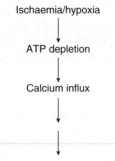

Ischaemia/hypoxia

↓

ATP depletion

↓

Calcium influx

↓

Oxygen free radical formation

There are a number of potential areas of therapeutic intervention arising from increased knowledge of the pathopysiological mechanisms of brain-cell injury during asphyxia.

Q. OK, quickly tell me about some of them.

A number of these potential therapies have been investigated, most significantly in the laboratory, to a lesser extent in adult stroke patients, and hardly at all in asphyxiated neonates:

— *magnesium* — regulatory role in 'gating' the NMDA channel
— *xanthine oxidase inhibitors* (allopurinol, oxypurinol) — reduce the production of oxygen free radicals
— *poly (ADP-ribose) polymerase (PARP) inhibitors* — excessive PARP activity can deplete energy sources
— *nitric-oxide synthase inhibitors* — the neurotoxic effects of glutamate are probably mediated by increased production of nitric oxide
— *antioxidants* and *free radical scavengers* — superoxide dismutase, catalase, lazaroids
— hypothermia — ? results in decreased energy use, reduced free-radical production, reduced excitatory amino acid toxicity, or other mechanisms

Q. How are you going to manage a baby that has been asphyxiated at birth?

Minimising brain injury requires careful attention to oxygen and glucose supplies. Autoregulation of cerebral blood flow is impaired in asphyxiated babies and cerebral perfusion is dependent on the maintenance of adequate systemic blood pressure. Treatment of pyrexia and fits are essential to minimise the metabolic rate of the brain. First-line anticonvulsant therapy is phenobarbital, phenytoin can be added, and a continuous infusion of benzodiazepine (e.g clonazepam) should be initiated for resistant fits. Fluid intake should be restricted to minimise brain swelling. Asphyxial damage to other organs of the body will need consideration and possible treatment, e.g. liver failure (bleeding, jaundice, hypoglycaemia) and renal failure.

Generally, those with grade 1 HIE will have no neurological sequelae but those with grade 3 HIE will have severe neurological deficit if they survive.

Tip

- Be careful not to introduce something that you are not able to talk sensibly about. Therefore, do not mention ATP depletion, burst suppression on EEG etc. unless you can potentially go further if asked.

REFERENCES
Hammerman C, Kaplan M 1998 Ischemia and reperfusion injury. Clin Perinatol 25: 757–779
Robertson N J, Edwards A D 1998 Recent advances in developing neuroprotective strategies for perinatal asphyxia. Curr Opin Pediatr 10: 575–580

NEONATAL FITS

Q. You are called to see an infant on the special care baby unit who is having intermittent jerking of all limbs associated with desaturations. How would you manage this baby?

My *immediate management* would be as follows:

1. Oxygen — high flow facial oxygen.
2. Intravenous access — while inserting a drip I would take blood for U&E, Ca^{2+}, Mg^{2+}, glucose, blood cultures, and TORCH screen.
3. Drugs: I would give a loading dose of i.v. phenobarbital, followed by a loading dose of i.v. phenytoin under ECG control if the phenobarbital was unsuccessful. If the fit continued I would start an i.v. clonazepam infusion. I would monitor for respiratory depression and intubate and ventilate if necessary.

Investigations and further management

Once the fit had been terminated, I would undertake investigations to ascertain a cause, and instigate specific treatment if indicated:

a) *? Asphyxia*:
— history: Apgars, antenatal history, intrapartum history
— investigation: cranial ultrasound with Dopplers, consider MRI

b) *? Meningitis*:
— history: prolonged rupture of membranes, maternal pyrexia
— investigation: lumbar puncture
— treatment: high-dose broad-spectrum i.v. antibiotics (include anaerobic cover, *Klebsiella*, and *E. Coli*)

c) *? Metabolic*:
— investigation: Na^+, Ca^{2+}, Mg^{2+}, glucose, urine metabolic screen, serum lactate, ammonia ($\pm$ CSF lactate)
— treatment: treat immediately if abnormal as this may terminate the convulsion

d) *?Drug withdrawal*:
— History: maternal history of drug usage
— investigation: urine toxicology

The duration of anticonvulsant treatment depends on the cause of the fit. Once the convulsions have ceased I would withdraw one drug at a time over a period of several days. Long-term maintenance anticonvulsants may be required if convulsions recur.

It is important to discuss the implications of the convulsion with the parents. I would explain that the prognosis is unpredictable but that if the fit was short-lived and due to a transient metabolic disturbance then this would be reassuring. The clinical state of the child will also affect the outcome.

REFERENCE
Ramenghi L A et al 1996 Neonatal seizures: aetiology, management and prognosis. Curr Paediatr 6: 173–177

BREAKING BAD NEWS

Q. How would you break bad news to a family on the neonatal unit?

This is a common problem, and it is never easy. However, I have found that if I follow a few simple rules the situation can be easier to handle. Ideally, the most experienced person available should break any bad news although this often needs to be done in the middle of the night when the registrar is the most senior person in the hospital.

Occasionally, I have had to break bad news to parents whom I have just met for the first time. This is never ideal and is difficult for both the doctor and the parents. In all cases adequate *preparation* before seeing the family is essential. It is important not to overlook the sex of the child and refer to the baby as 'it' or, inexcusably, to get the sex wrong. If the child has a name, then this should be used. I would read both the medical and nursing notes to get as much information as possible about the child's progress to date, problems encountered, what the parents have been told about the prognosis, and details of the social situation. As part of my preparation I would ensure that a suitable room is available which has space for everyone to sit, is private, and where we will not be interrupted. Tissues should be provided in the room.

I would want to speak to both parents together and include another family member or friend if they wish. A nurse should be present — ideally one who knows the family well. This allows the family to talk to them about the news after the interview is complete. I would introduce myself to the family by name, including my position. I would aim to be gentle in my approach, while telling the news in a factual manner using uncomplicated language.

The family may be aware that the baby is seriously unwell and may have prepared questions to ask. This is often a good starting point for the discussion. It is essential to *listen carefully to the parents* and not to interrupt. In my experience I have found that the family often accepts the news very calmly initially, although some react with grief and anger. The natural instinct is to comfort the family — I think it does no harm for the parents to see our own emotional reaction, and physical contact may be appreciated.

It is easy to give the parents a lot of information at this interview, but much will be forgotten and a further meeting should be arranged.

When talking to the parents of a child with a visible abnormality that is not necessarily life-threatening, such as a baby with a cleft palate or Down's syndrome, I feel that it is helpful to show them the abnormalities one by one, rather than showing them the problems all at once. This allows them to adapt slowly. If an operation is likely to be required, 'before and after' photographs can be shown. Literature relevant to the disorder and information about support groups should also be given.

It is important after any discussion with parents to write a summary of what has been said in the patient's notes. This ensures that all staff are aware of what has been said to the parents, should further explanations be required.

MORBIDITY AND MORTALITY IN NEONATOLOGY

Q. What can you tell us about mortality and morbidity in infants admitted to the neonatal unit?

There have been significant improvements in neonatal intensive care over the past decade and this is reflected in the reduced mortality rate of preterm infants. Factors that have improved mortality rates include the introduction of *surfactant* and *antenatal corticosteroids* to reduce the severity of respiratory distress syndrome, and improvements in the equipment we use, such as modern *ventilators.* This has allowed the survival of extremely low birth weight babies at gestations down to 23 weeks.

The incidence of deaths in term infants has been reduced as a result of *antenatal diagnosis,* which has resulted in the termination of some infants whose condition (e.g. Patau's syndrome) is incompatible with life. There have also been changes in antenatal management of conditions such as group B streptococcal infection, so that antibiotics given prophylactically to the mother have reduced the incidence of fatal disease in the newborn. Surgical techniques for correction of conditions such as congenital heart disease and congenital diaphragmatic hernia have improved and antenatal diagnosis allows the infant to be born in a centre with appropriate expertise.

The *pattern of morbidity* in neonates is changing. Increased survival of extremely low birth weight (ELBW) and low birth weight (LBW) infants has caused an increase in conditions such as *chronic lung disease* and *neurodevelopmental disabilities*, including poor cognitive function, cerebral palsy, blindness and deafness. Studies have shown that ELBW infants have higher rates of *cognitive impairment* and behavioural problems, needing extra help at school, compared with normal birth weight children, in mid-childhood. Hospital readmissions in early childhood are also more common in infants born preterm, especially those with chronic lung disease.

Despite an increase in survival of ELBW infants, there has been a reduction in the incidence and severity of *retinopathy of prematurity*. However, infants of <28 weeks gestation or <1000 g are still at considerable risk of needing surgical treatment for this condition.

It is difficult to predict at birth which infants will suffer long-term complications. Physiology-based scoring systems have been developed and may be useful for comparison between neonatal intensive care units or countries, but are not very useful for prediction of prognosis in individual cases.

There is wide variation in the reported incidence of these complications in different centres. These variations in outcome between units are not fully explained. There is evidence to suggest that infants born in bigger units fare better, presumably as a result of extensive experience among nursing and medical staff, and consideration should be given to concentrating deliveries of at-risk infants in a smaller number of hospitals.

Cardiology and respiratory medicine

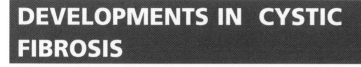

4

DEVELOPMENTS IN CYSTIC FIBROSIS

Q. There is more than one way to skin a cat — tell me about some of the controversies surrounding the management of cystic fibrosis!

Up until the last few years, individual paediatricians have looked after small numbers of children with cystic fibrosis (CF) on a full-time basis in their own hospital. More recently there has been a tendency to centralise care, either on a full-time or shared-care basis. With shared-care the children have at least an annual review in the tertiary centre for CF, where all aspects of care, including diet, physiotherapy, and medical care are reviewed. Although this centralisation necessitates the children having to travel greater distances, there are a number of benefits of this system:

— a more unified method of management
— access to dedicated CF dieticians, physiotherapists, and social workers
— participation in clinical research
— the development of regional expertise in the management of CF

There are a number of controversies about the treatment of CF. These include: the value of screening; the use of prophylactic antibiotics, deoxyribonuclease treatment; and the treatment of *Pseudomonas aeruginosa*.

Screening for CF
Current neonatal screening programmes in the UK, using the Guthrie card, incorporate the immunoreactive trypsin (IRT) assay in about 50% of newborn babies tested (Yorkshire, Gwent, Trent, Norfolk, Wales and other regions). If this is high (3 standard deviations above the mean), it is followed up by a repeat IRT and a search for the more common genetic mutations for CF using the original Guthrie card blood spot. If this second IRT value is high, sweat testing should then be offered, regardless of the genetic mutations search.

There is no doubt that screening results in earlier diagnosis of CF, conferring a number of potential *benefits*:

— earlier initiation of treatment (which may or may not confer long-term benefit for lung function and nutrition)
— prevention of unnecessary and inappropriate investigation, admission to hospital, and potential treatment of infants with CF wrongly assumed to have other pathologies, or while the diagnosis is being made
— genetic counselling for the parents

There are, however certain *disadvantages* to this screening programme:

— false positive results: the majority of infants with a high IRT on initial testing will not have CF. This creates unnecessary anxiety for parents with a normal child awaiting the second IRT result and possible sweat test
— the detection of carriers for CF — do you tell the parents that their child is a carrier?
— the detection of children with very mild disease who may not require the full gamut of available treatments. A proportion of well men attending infertility clinics have congenital bilateral absence of the vas deferens (CBAVD) and on testing are found to have two recognised genetic mutations for CF. Should we condemn them to twice-daily physiotherapy, altered diet and possible discrimination for health insurance, to name but a few of the problems of having CF?

Although many of the criteria for screening are not fulfilled (see page 269), screening for CF is becoming an accepted practice in the UK and overseas.

Antibiotic prophylaxis

The argument in favour of antistaphylococcal prophylaxis at the time of diagnosis is that *Staphylococcus aureus* can sometimes be isolated from bronchial secretions in children with CF from early infancy. This infection can be associated with inflammation, symptoms, and the development of lung damage. Arguments against prophylaxis include:

— side-effects of antibiotics — oral thrush, diarrhoea
— expense — £200 per year for flucloxacillin prophylaxis
— inconvenience — q.i.d. administration
— emergence of multiresistant organisms, e.g. MRSA
— ? predisposition to the acquisition of lung colonisation by other organisms, e.g. *Pseudomonas aeruginosa*

A recent Cochrane Review found that prophylactic flucloxacillin did reduce the prevalence of *S. aureus* in respiratory secretions in children with CF. It also reported a reduction in hospital admission with respiratory exacerbations in the first 2 years of life. However, it did not show any differences in lung function — although the follow-up duration of the studies included in the analysis was short and lung function measurement in young children is fraught with difficulties!

Deoxyribonuclease

Neutrophils release DNA when they die, causing increased viscosity of respiratory secretions in endobronchial infection. Human recombinant DNAse can be administered via a nebuliser to break down thickened secretions and promote mucociliary clearance. It is an expensive treatment, costing around £8 000 per year. For those children without significant airway disease, DNAse is therefore possibly not cost-effective. For those with significant disease (e.g. $FEV_1 < 60–75\%$) and symptoms, it may be worthwhile to give a trial of DNAse and observe its effect. In those who demonstrate an improvement in their lung function (>10% rise in FEV_1) and a reduction in symptoms it may be considered worthwhile to continue its use. The evidence for long-term use of DNAse, however, is not yet available. A recent Cochrane Review reported an improvement in lung function with 6 months' use, but there was no identifiable reduction in respiratory exacerbations or mortality. Longer-term studies are required to evaluate prolonged administration.

Treatment of *Pseudomonas aeruginosa*

Work originating from Denmark advocates the early and aggressive treatment of *Pseudomonas aeruginosa* (PA) if isolated from respiratory secretions of children with CF. This is because infection with PA is associated with increased and progressive deterioration in lung function. However, isolation of PA from a cough swab, sputum culture, or, to a lesser extent, bronchoalveolar lavage (BAL) does not necessarily equate with endobronchial infection. A recent paper investigating children under 5 years of age with CF found that the specificity and negative predictive value of oropharyngeal culture for PA was high, but that the sensitivity and positive predictive value was poor. In other words, if PA is isolated from sputum culture it may not mean that there is infection of the lower respiratory tract, but if it is *not* found on sputum culture it is likely that PA would not be isolated from BAL fluid. How hard one looks for PA colonisation is therefore relevant to the argument. Studies are under way randomising newly diagnosed infants to either bronchoscopy in the first 6 months of life, followed by repeated bronchoscopy with symptoms, or the more usual monitoring with sputum culture.

What should be done with a positive culture for PA is not clear. A one-off positive result may indicate colonisation rather than infection and it may not be repeated in subsequent cultures. Some would adopt the 'watch and wait' approach, whereas other centres would advocate high-dose oral ciprofloxacin and nebulised Colomycin on initial isolation of the organism to maximise the chance of eradication. Multicentre randomised controlled trials are required to ascertain the ideal approach to management.

Q. Tell us about the influence of molecular genetics on the treatment of CF.

Over 850 genetic mutations, resulting in an abnormality of the cystic fibrosis transmembrane regulator (CFTR) development or function, have been found to date. These mutations are classified into five groups according to their effect on the CFTR:

Class I — defective synthesis of the CFTR
Class II — inappropriate location of the CFTR within the cell
Class III —·defective CFTR regulation/activation
Class IV — partial function of the CFTR arising from altered chloride conduction characteristics
Class V — severe reduction in the normal CFTR protein as a result of aberrant mRNA splicing

Treatments, rather than a cure, could conceivably be tailored to the class of CFTR abnormality a child with CF demonstrates. For example, aerolised gentamicin may promote full-length CFTR mRNA production in those with class I mutations. Class II mutations (including ΔF508) result in trafficking defects in which the CFTR protein, synthesised in the endoplasmic reticulum, is not transported to the plasma membrane. Chemical 'chaperones', such as glycerol, are being investigated. Class III mutations, including G551D, resulting in pancreatic insufficiency and severe disease, have as yet not been amenable to pharmacological interventions in vitro. Class IV mutations, including R117H, associated with pancreatic sufficiency and mild disease, may be responsive to activation of the chloride channels. In vitro studies using milrinone, a phosphodiesterase inhibitor used in postoperative cardiac surgery as an inotropic agent, have shown promise. Repair of class V mutations is likely to involve stimulation of CFTR mRNA production, although I am not aware of any advances in this area.

Somatic gene therapy, incorporating the normal CFTR gene into the abnormal cells has undergone significant research both in vitro and in vivo. I know that phase III trials, applying CFTR-cDNA/adenovirus recombinants to the nasal and bronchial epithelia have taken place, particularly in the USA, but I am not sure how successful they have been.

Tips

● There is nothing like a controversial subject to keep you talking for 10 minutes. The good thing is that there are no right or wrong answers and you can quite happily sit on the fence. Do not blow it by being dogmatic about the way *your* centre treats CF being the only way.

● It is not a bad idea to say 'I am not aware of any research in this area . . .' or 'I am not sure of the latest developments . . .' You never know, you may strike gold, with the examiner telling *you* all about his pet subject or demonstrating his superior knowledge. Sit back and watch the seconds and minutes go by!

REFERENCES

Kearney C E, Wallis C E 2000 Deoxyribonuclease for cystic fibrosis (Cochrane Review). In: The Cochrane Library, Issue 1. Update software, Oxford.

Rubenstein R C, Zeitlin P L 1998 Use of protein repair therapy in the treatment of cystic fibrosis. Curr Opin Pediatr 10: 250–255

Scotet V, de Braekeleer M, Roussey M et al 2000 Neonatal screening for cystic fibrosis in Brittany, France: assessment of 10 years' experience and impact on prenatal diagnosis. Lancet 356: 789–794

Smyth A, Walters S 2000 Prophylactic antibiotics for cystic fibrosis (Cochrane Review). In: The Cochrane Library, Issue 1. Update Software, Oxford

ASTHMA

Q. Where do leukotriene receptor antagonists fit into the British Thoracic Society guidelines for the management of asthma in children?

At the present time the guidelines do not incorporate leukotriene receptor antagonists (LTRAs) into the step system (see page 38). This is because they (zafirlukast and montelukast) have only been introduced onto the market after the National Asthma Campaign guidelines were drawn up. Their role, particularly in children, has yet to be fully established. However, montelukast does have approval in Europe as a second-line 'controller' at step 3 or above in children aged 3 years and above. In other words, it should be considered as add-on therapy to inhaled corticosteroids instead of long-acting β_2 agonists. Zafirlukast has approved use at step 2 or above as a first-line 'preventer' in children aged 7 years and above (i.e. instead of low-dose inhaled cortico-steroids).

Montelukast has also been approved as monotherapy for prophylaxis in exercise-induced asthma. As more research is undertaken, particularly ran-domised controlled trials comparing leukotriene antagonists with low-dose inhaled corticosteroids, the indications for LTRAs may change significantly.

Q. How do leukotriene antagonists work?

The cysteinyl-leukotrienes (LTC_4, D_4 and E_4) are potent bronchoconstrictors, 100 to 1000 times more potent than histamine, producing airway narrowing even in non-asthmatic subjects. The leukotrienes are also more potent than prostaglandins and histamine in their ability to produce airway mucus. Inhaled LTD_4 and E_4 increase vascular permeability and cellular influx

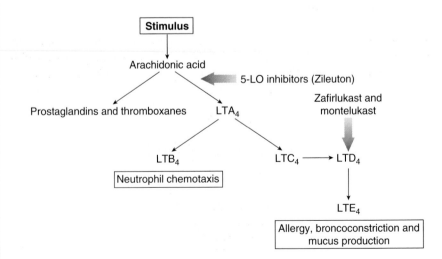

(eosinophils and neutrophils) in asthmatics, thereby amplifying inflammation. The leukotriene antagonists therefore have a role in reducing bronchoconstriction, decreasing airway mucus production, and down-regulating the inflammatory response.

LTE_4 is excreted in the urine and can be used as a marker of total cysteinyl-leukotriene production. Elevated levels are found in acute and chronic asthma, exercise-induced bronchospasm and following allergen challenge. LTE_4 synthase is found in eosinophils, mast cells and alveolar macrophages. LTB_4 is produced by macrophages, monocytes and neutrophils.

Q. Do you have any reservations about their use in children?

Data collected from patients involved in clinical trials of LTRAs suggest that they have an excellent safety profile. Their main advantages are that they are taken orally and their rapid onset of action (1–3 hours), both of which are likely to enhance compliance.

Commonly reported side-effects include headache, nausea, diarrhoea and transient liver dysfunction, but they appear no more frequently than in patients taking placebo. There have been several case reports in the adult literature of Churg-Strauss syndrome in patients taking both zafirlukast and montelukast. However, the consensus of opinion is that these were clinically unrecognised cases that became apparent on a tapering of the steroid dose after starting LTRAs. Caution should therefore be exercised in reducing steroid dosage of steroid-dependent asthmatics, checking for a rising peripheral eosinophil count.

Both zafirlukast and montelukast are metabolised by the cytochrome P450 system in the liver and caution should be taken when prescribing other medications metabolised in this way (e.g. warfarin, phenytoin, carbamazepine, cisapride). It is recommended that liver function should be checked periodically.

Q. Is asthma an inherited condition?

There is a great deal of evidence that asthma is a heritable condition. There is an increased prevalence of asthma in relatives of asthmatic subjects compared with those of non-asthmatics. Twin studies also demonstrate a significant increase in

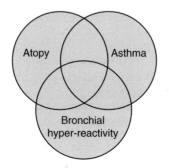

concordance among monozygotic compared with dizygotic twins. However, the interaction between genetic and environmental factors in the pathogenesis and development of the disease is of fundamental importance. Most asthmatics are atopic and demonstrate bronchial hyper-reactivity, but each of these features can occur without the other. It is likely that antigenic exposure in early life (or even in utero) can lead to asthma in those with a genetic predisposition.

Genetic studies have identified the gene loci for many of the factors involved in allergic, inflammatory and bronchoconstrictor responses seen in asthma, for example:

Chromosome 5   IL3, 4, 5, 9 and 13, LTC_4
Chromosome 6 $TNF\alpha$
Chromosome 12 $INF\gamma$

Candidate genes on chromosomes 7, 13, 14, 16 and 17 have also been implicated. Although there have been significant advances in the understanding of the heritability of asthma, no genes have been identified with any certainty. Ongoing worldwide collaborative research may one day give us the definitive answer to your question!

Key points

▲ LTRAs are the first new type of asthma drug in over 30 years.

▲ They produce bronchodilation, decrease mucus production, and diminish the inflammatory response, giving them a role as both reliever and preventer in asthma treatment.

▲ Urinary excretion of LTE_4 gives a means of monitoring the state of the body's inflammatory response.

▲ The LTRAs have approval for use in children > 3 years of age (montelukast) and > 7 years (zafirlukast), but at present are not incorporated into the National Asthma Campaign / British Thoracic Society guidelines.

▲ The genetics of asthma is yet to be clarified.

Tip

● If you are a budding molecular biologist the world is your oyster with this last question. Off you go into the incomprehensible language of candidate genes, genomic scanning, positional cloning, linkage studies, polymorphisms etc. For us mere mortals our advice is to stick to the 'basics' of genes and chromosomes!

REFERENCES

Holloway J W, Beghé B, Holgate S T 1999 The genetic basis of atopic asthma. Clin Exp Allergy 29: 1023–1032

Lipworth B J 1999 Leukotriene-receptor antagonists. Lancet 353: 57–62

Sandford A J, Paré P D 2000 The genetics of asthma. Am J Respir Crit Care Med 161: S202–S206

Weisberg S C 2000 Pharmacotherapy of asthma in children, with special reference to leukotriene-receptor antagonists. Pediatr Pulmonol 29: 46–61

BRONCHIOLITIS

Q. Tell me about bronchiolitis.

Bronchiolitis is an acute inflammatory respiratory illness of infancy characterised by tachypnoea, increased work of breathing, cough, +/- fever. It has a seasonal distribution, occurring primarily in the winter months in the UK and its peak incidence is in the 2 to 5 months age range.

A number of viral pathogens are implicated, the major culprit being the respiratory syncytial virus (RSV). Sixty percent of infants will have serological evidence of infection with RSV by their first birthday, rising to 95% by the age of 2. One to two percent of all infants will be admitted to hospital with bronchiolitis, the vast majority having a self-limiting illness of short duration. The mortality rate for those admitted to hospital is between 1% and 4%. However, up to 50–70% will have postbronchiolitic cough and wheeze and its relationship to the development of asthma has been highly researched.

Q. Tell me how you would treat it.

As already stated, bronchiolitis is a self-limiting condition. For those admitted to hospital, good nursing care, supplemental oxygen to maintain saturations and enteral/parenteral fluid and nutritional support are the mainstay of treatment. A wide range of other therapies are often given without any significant evidence for their effectiveness. These include β_2-agonists, ipratropium bromide, theophylline and corticosteroids (particularly in the USA where the definition of bronchiolitis includes the presence of wheeze). Nebulised adrenaline may offer short-term benefit, although the evidence for this is limited.

Q. Would you (or do you) use any of these medications to treat bronchiolitis?

Some would argue in favour of giving an infant with bronchiolitis and significant respiratory distress a one-off trial of nebulised β_2-agonist. In my experience I have found this to be unhelpful and in some infants it can actually cause a deterioration in their clinical status. I therefore do not carry out this practice, nor do I advocate the administration of ipratropium bromide or corticosteroids.

Ribavarin, an aerolised antiviral agent, has been given previously in the UK, especially to those infants at risk of more severe disease (premature infants, or those with congenital heart disease, bronchopulmonary dysplasia, or immunodeficiency). However, in the hospitals I have worked at, I have never seen it given. This is because it is expensive, labour-intensive in its administration (12–18 hours continuous aerosol for 3 days), there are concerns about its safety, and it is of questionable benefit.

Q. OK, so we cannot treat it — in what ways can we prevent bronchiolitis?

Ten to thirty percent of all cases of bronchiolitis in hospital are caused by cross-contamination. Although not proven, it is likely that doctors are the major culprits in passing the infection from one infant to another by not employing effective hand-washing procedures!

Rapid detection of virus on admission to hospital (by immunofluorescence) and segregation of infants who are positive for RSV may reduce the risk of cross-infection.

Passive immunisation

Several large multicentre international studies have investigated the benefit of passive immunisation with polyclonal RSV hyperimmune globulin and monoclonal antibody in preventing RSV hospitalisation. These studies have targeted those infants born prematurely (≤35 weeks gestation) and/or those with bronchopulmonary dysplasia. The PREVENT study showed a 41% reduction and the IMpact-RSV study a 55% reduction in hospitalisation from RSV infection. A recent Cochrane Review reported that RSV hyperimmune globulin is effective, with 17 and 50 patients treated to prevent one hospitalisation and one ICU admission respectively. The mortality rate from RSV bronchiolitis is very low and unaffected by passive immunisation. It must be remembered, however, that this form of prevention is very expensive and labour-intensive, requiring 5 monthly injections. It is only appropriate for those infants likely to have significant disease.

Active immunisation

The first attempts at vaccinating infants and children against RSV infection in the 1960s used a formalin-inactivated preparation. It failed on two accounts, firstly in not protecting the children against naturally acquired RSV infection, but also because it resulted in more serious RSV lower-respiratory-tract disease in the subsequent season. Since then recombinant, subunit, live and attenuated vaccines have all been developed and tested in animals and in some cases, healthy adult volunteers and children with cystic fibrosis. Some of these vaccines show promise in that the recipients develop RSV antibodies, but they have yet to be tested in infancy.

Tip

● What a gift of a question! No excuses here for not talking 'until the cows come home' about something that all of us have had significant clinical exposure to. You can direct the subject towards the conundrum of the association between bronchiolitis and asthma; allergen avoidance and the hygeine hypothesis; the change in family dynamics over the last 20 years with the loss of the extended family and a resultant reduction in viral exposure in children's early years, etc. etc. Talk until the examiners tell you to shut up, or they nod off.

REFERENCES

IMpact-RSV Study Group 1998 Palivizumab, a humanized respiratory syncytial virus monoclonal antibody, reduces hospitalization from respiratory syncytial virus infection in high-risk infants. Pediatrics 102: 531–537

Kneyber M C J, Moll M A, de Groot R 2000 Treatment and prevention of respiratory syncytial virus infection. Eur J Paediatr 159: 399–411

PREVENT Study Group 1997 Reduction of respiratory syncytial virus hospitalization among premature infants with bronchopulmonary dysplasia using respiratory syncytial virus immune globulin prophylaxis. Pediatrics 99: 93–99

Wang E E L, Tang N K 2000 Immunoglobulin for preventing respiratory syncytial virus infection (Cochrane Review). In: The Cochrane Library, Issue 1. Update Software, Oxford

PERSISTENT COUGH

Q. What possible diagnoses go through your mind when you see a child with persistent cough?

First of all, it is important to define what is meant by persistent cough — my understanding is that any child having daily cough for at least 3 weeks can be described as having persistent symptoms. The second important aspect is the nature of the cough. A *productive, moist cough* is almost certainly abnormal and an underlying pathology must be sought. Potential diagnoses in this category of cough include:

— cystic fibrosis
— inhalation of a foreign body
— primary ciliary dyskinesia
— immunodeficiency and bronchiectasis
— congenital lung pathology e.g. tracheo/bronchomalacia, vascular ring

The more common situation is of a child with a *persistent unproductive cough*, referred to the outpatient department by the general practitioner, who is frustrated by the continued symptoms despite a number of pharmacological interventions. The list of potential diagnoses here is very different from the one above:

— post-infectious cough — bronchiolitis, whooping cough, mycoplasma
— cough receptor sensitivity (CRS)
— cough variant asthma (CVA)
— psychogenic cough
— gastro-oesophageal reflux (+/− chronic aspiration)
— tuberculosis

Differentiating between the possible causes for the child's symptoms can be very difficult, particularly because detailed investigation may be very unrewarding. However, I would investigate all children with persistent unproductive cough by means of chest X-ray and baseline spirometry in those old enough to do it. This will, in the majority of cases, rule out significant pathology and give an assessment of lung function. Except for gastro-oesophageal reflux, TB and aspiration, both chest X-ray and spirometry are likely to be completely normal.

Q. Tell me about cough receptor sensitivity and cough variant asthma.

Cough receptors/sensory nerves are located in and under the epithelial surface lining the airways (rapidly adapting fibres — Aδ myelinated fibres, and bronchial C fibres — non-myelinated afferents) and possibly in the alveolar wall (pulmonary C fibres). Mechanical (dust, foreign body, mucus), chemical (nicotine, citric acid), and inflammatory (histamine, bradykinin) mediators stimulate these receptors, which pass signals via the vagus nerve to the 'cough centre' in the brainstem. Efferent nerves to the glottis, muscles of expiration and pelvic floor then initiate a cough. Cortical function can modulate the cough via its effects on the cough centre. Disruption of the airway epithelium by whatever means, including cough itself, can lead to further sensitisation of the airways, producing increased cough receptor sensitivity.

Cough variant asthma is a term, first coined in the early 1980s, used to describe those children (and adults) labelled as having 'asthma' with cough as their primary and only symptom, without a demonstrable wheezy component. The prevalence of asthma has risen exponentially over the last two decades and to a large extent this is because of children and adults being labelled as cough variant asthmatics. As with many aspects of medicine, there is controversy, with proponents of CVA advocating that children with cough alone should be treated as having asthma, and detractors stating that a child with asthma must have a wheezy component. To date, I am unaware of any published placebo-controlled trials on the benefits of asthma medication in children with cough alone.

Q. What can we treat persistent cough in children with then?

The most important thing is to exclude underlying pathology, as mentioned previously, with chest X-ray +/– spirometry as a minimum. Reassurance and explanation of the mechanisms of cough may be all that is then necessary. Fortunately, in the majority of cases there will be a spontaneous reduction in cough severity over a period of weeks (or even months) — the period effect. There is a significant number of anti-tussive medications, (over 200 listed in the British National Formulary) available 'over-the-counter' for the treatment of cough. Although I am not aware of the figure for the UK, I know that in the USA approximately $2 billion and in Australia $125 million is spent per year on cough and cold remedies.

Anecdotal evidence for the effectiveness of nebulised lignocaine in CRS exists. Similarly, anecdotal and non-placebo-controlled trials report the benefit of cough suppressants (codeine, pholcodeine), antihistamines, decongestants, and combination medications in the treatment of persistent cough. There are, however, very few randomised placebo-controlled studies of the use of cough medications in children and none demonstrate statistically significant benefit for cough medications over placebo. However, persistent cough can cause family distress and so if a cough medication is deemed necessary, a simple cough linctus should suffice. It is important to bear in mind that many of the cough medications have significant side-effects in overdosage (and even at pharmacological doses).

For cough that is thought to be psychogenic in origin, or with a significant psychological component, breathing techniques to try and suppress cough may be beneficial.

Tip

● You may be asked specifically if you think CVA is a separate clinical entity within the umbrella term of 'asthma'. This is a difficult question! The vast majority of children with asthma will wheeze if given the right stimulus (exercise, viral infection, exposure to allergens, methacholine challenge!). Asking a child (who is old enough) to keep a peak flow diary over a number of weeks may demonstrate significant variability consistent with a diagnosis of asthma, even if audible wheeze has never been heard by the parents or paediatrician.

REFERENCES

Chang A B 1999 Cough, cough receptors, and asthma in children. Pediatr Pulmonol 28: 59–70

Chang A B, Robertson C F 2000 Cough in children. Med J Aust 172: 122–125

Cough medication in children. (1999). Drug Ther Bull 37: 19–21

CARDIOMYOPATHY

Q. What can you tell me about the types of cardiomyopathy in children?

Cardiomyopathies are structural and functional diseases of the myocardium and may be primary or secondary. Primary cardiomyopathies include dilated, hypertrophic and restrictive forms. Secondary causes of cardiomyopathy include: viral, bacterial, and fungal infections; storage disorders (glycogen storage disorders, mucopolysaccharidoses); musculoskeletal disorders (muscular dystrophy, myopathies); and drugs (anthracyclines).

Q. Tell me more about dilated, hypertrophic and restrictive cardiomyopathies.

Dilated cardiomyopathy

Dilated cardiomyopathy (DCM) has a familial incidence in 30–40% of cases. The most common inheritance pattern is autosomal dominant, although autosomal recessive and X-linked patterns have been described. Nutritional and environmental factors are also thought to be important. Patients have biventricular dilatation and usually present with congestive cardiac failure. Examination may reveal tachypnoea, tachycardia, a displaced apex beat, mitral regurgitation and hepatomegaly. A chest X-ray may show cardiomegaly and pulmonary venous congestion. The diagnosis can usually be confirmed by echocardiography. *Treatment* is divided into medical and surgical: medical treatment is directed at relief of heart failure using diuretics, inotropes and oral vasodilators; some children may require cardiac transplantation. One-third of children with DCM die, one-third make a complete recovery, and one-third improve but continue to have cardiac dysfunction.

Hypertrophic cardiomyopathy

Hypertrophic cardiomyopathy (HCM) is characterised by asymmetric left ventricular and intraventricular septal hypertrophy. The left ventricle is not dilated and there is usually outflow tract obstruction. It is inherited as an autosomal dominant trait with variable penetrance. Numerous genes, all encoding sarcoplasmic proteins, have been isolated. It may also be inherited as a maternally-inherited mitochondrial disorder. Presenting complaints include chest pain, palpitations and syncope. A small percentage of patients present with sudden death following exercise. A chest X-ray will reveal cardiomegaly, but the diagnosis is confirmed by echocardiography. The *medical treatment* of choice for symptomatic children is β-blockers, but calcium channel blockers are also used. Symptomatic arrhythmias should be treated with amiodarone. *Surgical intervention* is indicated in patients with obstructive symptoms. Left ventricle myomyectomy (Morrow operation) has been shown to prolong life and provide symptomatic relief in some centres. Patients with HCM should be given antibiotic prophylaxis against endocarditis.

Restrictive cardiomyopathy

Restrictive cardiomyopathy is characterised by deposits within the myocardium. The most common causes in children are endomyocardial fibroelastosis (EMF) and Loeffler's EMF, which is associated with eosinophilia.

REFERENCE

Gajarski R J, Towbin J A 1995 Recent advances in the etiology, diagnosis, and treatment of myocarditis and cardiomyopathies in children. Curr Opin Pediatr 7: 587–594

PRIMARY CILIARY DYSKINESIA

Q. Tell me about primary ciliary dyskinesia.

Primary ciliary dyskinesia (PCD) is a global term used to describe a group of conditions in which there is a congenital defect in the structure and/or function of cilia. Included in the group is Kartagener's syndrome (situs inversus, sinusitis and bronchiectasis), which accounts for around 50% of cases. The remainder have situs solitus but cilial abnormalities — the immotile cilia syndrome is one of these.

The incidence of PCD is not known but it is likely to be around 1 in 15 000 to 1 in 20 000 of the Caucasian population in the UK. This should mean around 70 new cases a year and a cohort of about 3000 patients in total. However, the known incidence is far less than this, with only about 150 known cases. The explanation for this is that some children and adults with recurrent sinopulmonary disease are not being diagnosed correctly.

Q. OK, how do you make the diagnosis?

Because there are no definitive diagnostic features for PCD, diagnosis relies on laboratory investigation. A child with dextrocardia, situs inversus or recurrent sinopulmonary disease warrants investigation.

An initial screening test is the *saccharin test*. A tablet of saccharin is placed onto the inferior nasal turbinate and the time taken for the person to taste saccharin is recorded. With normal nasal mucociliary clearance, tasting should be apparent by 60 minutes. For the test the patient must sit with the head forward, and must not sneeze, sniff, cough, eat, or drink. For all these reasons it is not suitable for younger children and uncooperative patients. If the test is negative (i.e. no taste within 60 minutes) and for the noncompliant patient, ciliary beat-frequency measurement is necessary. This requires nasal (or bronchial) brushings to obtain epithelial cells, which are examined under the microscope for the presence of functioning cilia. The patient must be free of upper respiratory tract infections for 4–6 weeks prior to the test. More detailed electron microscope analysis of the cilia may be necessary in a minority of patients to identify specific primary ultrastructural cilial abnormalities.

Q. How do you manage a child with PCD?

In many respects, management is the same as that for cystic fibrosis lung disease. Daily physiotherapy to promote mucociliary clearance is the mainstay of treatment. Aggressive treatment of respiratory exacerbations with antibiotics aims to delay progression of lung disease. Sinusitis, secretory otitis media, and persistent rhinitis occur frequently and may be resistant to more common interventions. Insertion of grommets may result in a continually discharging ear and should not be undertaken routinely.

Cardiology and respiratory medicine

A significant proportion will have subfertility or infertility and patients should be made aware of this at an appropriate age.

Tip

● This is a subject that you either know all about or you have never heard of! If it is the former, you could introduce it if asked to talk about an interesting patient you have seen recently. If you are in the latter group then admit complete ignorance and hope they move on. However, they may probe your knowledge by asking about Kartagener's syndrome or immotile cilia syndrome and expect you to expand upon this. Don't panic!

REFERENCES

Bush A, Cole P, Hariri M et al 1998 Primary ciliary dyskinesia: diagnosis and standards of care. Eur Respir J 12: 982–988

Meeks M, Bush A 2000 Primary ciliary dyskinesia (PCD). Pediatr Pulmonol 29: 307–316

HYPOPLASTIC LEFT HEART SYNDROME

Q. What can you tell us about the infant with hypoplastic left heart syndrome?

Hypoplastic left heart syndrome describes a spectrum of disorders with varying degrees of severity. Basically, it includes children who have left sided malformations of the heart which might include aortic atresia or stenosis, hypoplasia of the aortic arch and hypoplasia or absence of the left ventricle. It is the most common congenital cardiac anomaly causing death in infancy. There were no therapeutic options until relatively recently.

The condition is diagnosed antenatally in some women on a detailed scan. At present, antenatal diagnosis allows counselling, but no antenatal therapeutic intervention. After counselling, couples may feel that they would prefer termination of pregnancy because the risks are so high for the child. If the couple opt to continue the pregnancy, the child should be delivered in a centre with facilities available for specialist cardiac surgery if it is felt appropriate.

An infant with undiagnosed hypoplastic left heart syndrome may seem entirely normal at birth. They may then collapse when the ductus arteriosus closes, causing tachycardia, tachypnoea, pallor, or sometimes cyanosis. The child has cardiovascular shock with poorly palpable peripheral pulses and a metabolic acidosis. There may be no audible heart murmur. The differential diagnosis will include sepsis, which is obviously more common. Chest X-ray shows cardiomegaly and an ECG shows right ventricular hypertrophy, with low voltages over the left-sided chest leads.

Q. What is the physiology of hypoplastic left heart syndrome then?

The infant is dependent on the right ventricle supplying both pulmonary and systemic circulations. At birth the right ventricle supplies the aorta via the ductus arteriosus. Oxygenated blood returning from the lungs passes from the left atrium to the right atrium via the foramen ovale. When the ductus arteriosus closes or the pulmonary resistance falls after a few days, the right ventricle is unable to supply sufficient oxygenated blood to the systemic circulation.

At diagnosis, it is important to maintain patency of the ductus if possible, using prostaglandin E_1 (alprostadil). Then the aim should be to balance the pulmonary and systemic circulations. This can be done by manipulating oxygenation so that saturations are about 75–80%. This avoids pulmonary vasodilatation (when blood would 'pool' in the pulmonary vasculature, reducing systemic circulation). Alkalosis should be avoided and respiratory acidosis may help by maintaining a degree of pulmonary vasoconstriction.

Q. What surgical options are there?

Cardiac transplantation would be 'curative', but there are few donors of suitable hearts at this age, despite recent well-publicised cases of young children requiring transplants.

More realistically, it may be possible to do a series of operations, aiming to modify the circulation so that the right ventricle supplies both circulations. This is called the *Norwood procedure* and is palliative. The first stage is performed as soon as the baby is clinically stable. The aortic arch is reconstructed and redirected from the right ventricle. An atrial septostomy allows circulation of pulmonary venous blood to the right side of the heart — in other words replacing the patent foramen ovale. A modified Blalock-Taussig shunt is formed which allows blood flow from the subclavian artery to the pulmonary artery, guaranteeing pulmonary circulation. If the balance of pulmonary and systemic circulations can be maintained following the first stage procedure, two further stages of operation are performed when the infant is older in order to secure systemic venous return directly to the pulmonary artery using a modified Fontan procedure.

POSTOPERATIVE MANAGEMENT IN CARDIAC SURGERY

Q. What can you tell us about the postoperative care of a child who has had cardiac surgery?

Although I have not had the opportunity to work in a unit specialising in paediatric cardiac surgery, I know that there are some basic principles which should be followed.

Firstly, any child undergoing heart surgery should be cared for in a *specialist centre* where there are paediatric cardiac surgeons, cardiac anaesthetists, and a paediatric intensive care unit with considerable expertise.

Secondly, I would want to be familiar with the child undergoing the operation preoperatively, so that I was aware of the congenital defect, the operation planned, possible complications, and any *incidental medical conditions*. For example, many children with atrio-ventricular septal defects also have trisomy 21 and may have a tendency to upper airway obstruction. Some children with aortic arch problems may have DiGeorge syndrome, with a tendency to hypocalcaemia and T-cell lymphopenia.

Postoperatively, I would assess the child on the intensive care unit after a handover of information from the surgeon or anaesthetist. It is important to ensure that the child has adequate *analgesia* and *sedation*, particularly those children who have had high pulmonary vascular blood flow and are more at risk of reactive pulmonary hypertension.

I would keep a close eye on *fluid balance*, particularly in those children who have been on cardiopulmonary bypass as they are at risk of capillary leakage and will need fluid restriction. Loss into drains should be monitored, as this fluid may need to be replaced with whole blood. The child should be catheterised for accurate urine output assessment. I would give intravenous fluid including glucose, but be prepared for a high blood glucose level following cardiac bypass. Pulse, perfusion and blood pressure may be useful, but a central venous catheter will be most valuable for assessing fluid balance.

The child should have continuous *ECG monitoring* as cardiac arrhythmias, especially sinus tachycardia, are common postoperatively and may have important effects on cardiac output. The child will be at risk of hypokalaemia (precipitating arrhythmias), and hypocalcaemia, which reduces cardiac contractility following cardiac bypass. Electrolytes should be checked frequently and replaced via a central venous line. Many children will have temporary pacing wires inserted during the operation, which can be used in heart block or for overdrive pacing of tachyarrhythmias.

It is important to watch the child's *blood pressure* meticulously and this is usually possible via an intra-arterial line. The blood pressure may go up after an operation where there has been high preoperative left ventricular pressure, such as repair of coarctation of the aorta. This can be treated with vasodilators such as sodium nitroprusside and glyceryl trinitrate or with beta-blockers.

More commonly, the blood pressure falls postoperatively and may be associated with lactic acidosis related to underperfusion. This may be a sign of fluid depletion, particularly blood loss, when replacement of colloid should have a rapid effect. However, it may be a sign of impaired cardiac contractility, when it might be necessary to consider inotropic support.

Q. What inotropes might you use?

It depends mainly on the problem: infusion of calcium might have powerful inotropic effects if the blood calcium is low; in the same way, magnesium replacement may be valuable.

Dopamine is often used at relatively low doses when it stimulates adrenergic β_1-receptors, improving the contractility of the myocardium. It is also thought to improve blood flow to the renal and mesenteric vessels at low dose, thus ensuring adequate perfusion (which might have been impaired by the initial cardiac abnormality or by a perioperative drop in systemic blood pressure).

Dobutamine stimulates β_1- and β_2-receptors, increasing stroke volume and heart rate. It does not seem to increase pulmonary vascular resistance so may be useful when right ventricular function is compromised.

Adrenaline and *isoprenaline* are powerful inotropic agents and may be used if larger doses of dobutamine are required. Noradrenaline is most useful as a vasoconstrictor, so is less useful in the postoperative situation, unless sepsis is a factor affecting blood pressure.

Tip

● Don't be afraid to admit to limitations in your clinical experience — nobody knows everything. The examiners will still be impressed if you can demonstrate a practical approach to problem-solving.

KAWASAKI DISEASE

PASS ✓

Q. Tell me about Kawasaki disease.

Kawasaki disease, also known as acute febrile mucocutaneous lymph node syndrome, was first described in 1967 by Tomisaku Kawasaki of Japan. It is the commonest recognised cause of acquired heart disease in childhood in the developed world (rheumatic fever is the commonest in the developing world). The prevalence in the UK is about 170 new cases a year (3–4 cases per 100 000 <5-year-olds, compared with 90 cases per 100 000 <5-year-olds in Japan). The male to female ratio is up to 2:1 and 75% of cases occur in the under-5-years age group. The recurrence rate is up to 3%.

Q. What causes it?

The aetiology is unknown. During the early phases of the illness there is a marked activation of the immune system, with increased numbers of activated T and B cells, monocytes, macrophages, neutrophils, adhesion molecules, cytokines and interleukins. An infectious cause is likely, although no single agent has been identified with any consistency. This is supported by a seasonal pattern (highest incidence in winter/spring), occurrence of outbreaks and a higher incidence amongst siblings of affected individuals. Several associations have been described, including carpet shampoo, house-dust mite, *Proprionobacterium acnes*, parvovirus B19, EBV, other herpes viruses, and retroviruses. Recently a superantigenic pathogenesis has been postulated. The underlying pathological process is a diffuse vasculitis affecting small-and medium-sized blood vessels.

Q. How do you make the diagnosis?

Diagnosis is essentially clinical and relies on fever for at least 5 consecutive days, plus four out of five other criteria:

1. Bilateral non-exudative conjunctival injection.
2. Oral changes — swollen, erythematous or cracked lips, 'strawberry' tongue and mucosal hyperaemia.
3. Peripheral extremity changes — erythema, oedema, and desquamation of the hands and feet (desquamation is often a late feature, i.e. after 10 days).
4. Polymorphous rash.
5. Cervical lymphadenopathy — occurs in 50–70% and very often there may only be one enlarged, tender node >1.5 cm in diameter.

Patients with 'atypical' Kawasaki disease, who manifest fewer than four of the five features, are at risk of coronary artery aneurysm formation. Kawasaki disease should therefore always be considered in the differential diagnosis of prolonged fever, especially in infants. Other non-specific features described include irritability, aseptic meningitis, cough, diarrhoea and vomiting, urethritis, arthralgia and arthritis, gallbladder hydrops, and hepatic dysfunction. A useful clue to diagnosis that is sometimes seen is redness and induration at the site of a BCG scar.

It is necessary to exclude other diagnoses that can demonstrate some, most, or all of the above signs and symptoms by appropriate investigation. These include streptococcal and staphylococcal infections, leptospirosis, rickettsia infections, measles, and Stevens-Johnson syndrome.

Q. OK, you have made your diagnosis, how are you going to treat it?

Recommendations have been drawn together in a consensus statement from the Third International Kawasaki Disease Symposium. For effective treatment, diagnosis should be made within 10 days of onset of fever. The infant/child should receive:

1. Intravenous immunoglobulins — 2 g/kg over 8–12 hours.
2. High-dose aspirin — 80–100 mg/kg/day, given 6-hourly for 14 days or until the fever remits, then continued as a low dose, 3–5 mg/kg/day as a single dose, until cardiological assessment at 6–8 weeks.

The child requires initial cardiological investigation with ECG and echocardiography at presentation, looking for evidence of coronary artery dilatation, aneurysm formation, pericarditis, and myocarditis. This should be followed by repeat echocardiograms 2 and 8 weeks later. If normal at 8 weeks, it is highly unlikely that macroscopic dilatation will occur subsequently. Aspirin can be stopped at this point. If abnormalities persist, regular echocardiography should be carried out and low-dose aspirin continued.

Q. What is the prognosis for the condition?

Prior to immunoglobulin and aspirin therapy, the incidence of coronary artery aneurysm formation was in the order of 20–25%. Abnormalities are more likely in those with high thrombocytosis, leucocytosis, a younger age, male sex and prolonged fever. Interestingly, a major study in the UK suggested that immunoglobulin administration within the first 10 days of onset may not actually reduce this figure by a significant margin. However, its use does dramatically improve mortality. It may be that immunoglobulins and aspirin reduce the severity (i.e. the diameter of coronary aneurysms) and speed up the resolution of the aneurysms. Mortality in this country is 2–4% and death usually occurs within the first 3 months. Mortality in Japan is only around 0.08%. These huge differences in mortality rates may be due in part to the under treatment of the condition in the UK, but may also be because intravenous immunoglobulin is less effective in UK disease (? due to a different aetiology or because of a different donor population for immunoglobulin production). Those with persistent coronary artery dilatation require long-term follow-up with a paediatric cardiologist and, at an appropriate age, an adult cardiologist.

Key points

▲ The definitive diagnosis of Kawasaki disease is based on fever of 5 days' duration plus four of the five other criteria.

▲ Treatment consists of high dose immunoglobulin infusion (2 g/kg body weight) plus high dose aspirin (80–100 mg/kg/day in divided doses) in the acute phase, followed by low-dose aspirin (3–5 mg/kg/day as a single dose) until cardiological assessment 6 to 8 weeks after diagnosis.

Tip

● Kawasaki disease remains an old favourite of examiners. Fortunately, although there has been a great deal of speculation in the literature about its causation, diagnosis and management have essentially remained unchanged.

REFERENCES

Curtis N, Levin M 1998 Kawasaki disease thirty years on. Curr Opin Pediatr 10: 24–33

David T J (ed.) 1993 Recent advances in paediatrics 11. Churchill Livingstone, Edinburgh

Dhillon R et al 1993 Management of Kawasaki disease in the British Isles. Arch Dis Child 69: 631–638

Laupland K B Dele Davies H 1999 Epidemiology, etiology, and management of Kawasaki disease: state of the art. Pediatr Cardiol 20: 177–183

COMPLICATIONS OF CONGENITAL HEART DISEASE

Q. Tell me briefly about congenital heart disease.

Congenital heart disease (CHD) has an incidence of 8 per 1000 live births in the UK. Eight abnormalities account for 80% of CHD — VSD, ASD, PDA, tetralogy of Fallot, pulmonary stenosis, coarctation of the aorta, aortic stenosis, and transposition of the great arteries (TGA). With improving ultrasonography technology, the vast majority of cases of severe congenital heart disease are diagnosed antenatally. However, about 25–30% of cases are recognised in the first year of life — a significant proportion presenting in the first few weeks of life with cyanosis (TGA, pulmonary atresia/stenosis, tricuspid atresia) or heart failure (severe aortic stenosis, coarctation of aorta, hypoplastic left heart syndrome). The diagnosis may also be made following the detection of a heart murmur. Prompt recognition and appropriate treatment are essential for survival and maximal growth and development.

Q. What are some of the complications of congenital heart disease?

There are many complications of congenital heart disease, which are related to the underlying anatomy. These are best considered under the following headings:

a) *General.* Children with uncomplicated acyanotic obstructive heart lesions show a normal growth pattern and normal development. However, children with shunting of blood from left to right or from right to left sides of the heart show a growth pattern of weight and height delay proportional to the size of the shunt. Children with shunts have been shown to have delay in the acquisition of motor skills and those with right to left shunts have shown a significant lowering of IQ.

b) *Pulmonary hypertension.* Severe, prolonged pulmonary hypertension results in Eisenmenger's syndrome with reversed or bi-directional flow across the heart. Heart-lung transplantation is the only treatment in severe cases.

c) *Cardiac arrhythmia.* Supraventricular tachycardia occurs most frequently in children with structurally normal hearts, in adults with atrial septal defects, and in Ebstein's anomaly. Cardiac surgery can result in disruption or damage to the conducting system of the heart.

d) *Infective endocarditis.* This is an uncommon complication and is only associated with dental surgery in a minority of cases. It is difficult to diagnose but must be considered in any child with congenital heart disease with pyrexia of unknown origin.

e) *Thrombosis and embolism.* Cerebral vessel thrombosis is a rare but potentially disastrous complication of congenital heart disease. Children with cyanotic heart disease are hypercoagulable due to polycythaemia and this is exacerbated by dehydration. Therefore, there should be a lower threshold for treatment of gastroenteritis, pyrexia, and poor feeding than for a 'normal' child. Paradoxical embolism, secondary to detachment of mural thrombus from within the heart in cyanotic heart disease, and cerebral abscess formation are potentially life-threatening, though rare, complications.

f) *Sudden death.* Hypertrophic obstructive cardiomyopathy is associated with sudden death. All cardiac defects with left-sided obstruction are associated with collapse on exercise.

Q. You mentioned infective endocarditis. What advice would you give about antibiotic cover in children with congenital heart disease?

Good oral hygiene and regular dental check-ups are essential for all children with congenital heart disease. It is important that the family is educated about the importance of prophylaxis and passes this information to the dentist/physician caring for their child.

Prophylaxis for dental surgery:

1. Oral *amoxicillin* 1 hour prior to procedure:
   - <5 years old — 750 mg
   - 5–10 years old — 1.5 g
   - >10 years old — 3 g
2. For those who have received penicillin in last 4 weeks or who are allergic to penicillin, use *clindamycin*:
   - < 5 years old — 150 mg
   - 5–10 years old — 300 mg
   - > 10 years old — 600 mg

Gastroenterology and infection

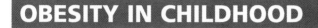

OBESITY IN CHILDHOOD

Q. What can you tell me about obesity in childhood?

Obesity is a problem seen quite frequently in outpatient clinics. It is becoming increasingly common in the populations of developed countries. This is most likely to be due to reduced energy expenditure — children are doing less exercise (particularly traditional daily activities such as walking to school) and have more sedentary pastimes, such as watching television and playing computer games. Excessive eating is also a trend, particularly with increased availability of convenience food. The importance of obesity is the increased risk of cardiovascular disease and diabetes in adult life.

Most children we see have '*simple obesity*', the result of an imbalance between energy input and output. However, there are other causes of obesity which should be considered, as there may be effective treatments. A variety of *endocrine diseases* cause obesity, for example hypothyroidism, Cushing's syndrome, hypogonadism, and hypothalamic and hypopituitary disorders. Usually, these can be distinguished from simple obesity by the history and examination, especially growth data. Obese children with endocrine disorders are usually short, whereas children with simple obesity tend to be taller than expected.

Children may be obese as a result of *medication*, for example steroid use (although those on long-term steroids are usually aware of this potential side-effect). Other children may be obese as a result of immobility, for example children with spina bifida.

Genetic causes of obesity include Down's syndrome, and Prader Willi syndrome, where children have an uncontrollable appetite. *Congenital leptin deficiency* also causes severe, early onset of obesity and hyperphagia during infancy.

Q. So, what can you tell us about leptin deficiency?

This has been described fairly recently. Leptin is a hormone which is the gene product of the *ob* gene. It is thought to act by regulating adipose tissue mass through hypothalamic effects on satiety and energy expenditure. Leptin levels have been found to be high in people with simple obesity, a finding which is thought to be due to leptin resistance.

So far, leptin has been studied mainly in obese mice, but also in humans deficiency seems to be associated with severe obesity and hypogonadotrophic hypogonadism. It is possible to treat leptin deficient patients, giving replacement therapy, with good effect on weight reduction.

RECURRENT ABDOMINAL PAIN

Q. What do you know about recurrent abdominal pain?

Recurrent abdominal pain (RAP) is a common childhood complaint that I have encountered many times in the clinic. It is evenly distributed between the sexes and social classes and is relatively common, with an incidence of approximately 10% in children over 5 years old. An organic cause is found in less than 10% of these.

The *organic causes* of recurrent abdominal pain are:

1. *Gastrointestinal* — gastro-oesophageal reflux, gastritis/duodenitis, constipation, inflammatory bowel disease, coeliac disease, gallstones
2. *Urological* — recurrent UTIs, reflux nephropathy, renal stones
3. *Haematological* — abdominal crisis in sickle cell disease, hypersplenism
4. *Miscellaneous* — porphyria, Henoch-Schönlein-purpura, lead poisoning

The incidence of RAP is highest between 5 and 7 years and between 12 and 14 years. The pain described is typically periumbilical and sharp and colicky in nature. The frequency of pain varies from child to child but, in order to fulfil the diagnosis of RAP, there should be at least three separate episodes within a 3-month period, severe enough to affect the child's activities. The pain does not usually wake the child at night and there is no relationship to eating, activity, or bowel habits. The children often have other somatic complaints and there is an association with school refusal. Physical examination and investigations are normal.

Q. How would you manage a child with recurrent abdominal pain?

It is important during the first consultation to obtain a picture regarding the nature of the pain, the degree of disruption the pain causes, and how the pain is dealt with by the patient, family and school.

Key questions to be asked initially would be:

a) *Location of the pain?* Periumbilical pain suggests a non-organic cause, whereas epigastric, suprapubic, or lateral pain is more likely to be of organic origin.
b) *Timing of the pain?* Post-prandial pain suggests dyspepsia or constipation. Nocturnal pain suggests duodenitis/duodenal ulceration. Pain starting on Monday mornings (school phobia), pain starting on the death of a pet, moving home or school, divorce or death of a parent, or a stepfather moving in (when one should consider sexual abuse) all suggest a non-organic cause.
c) *Any change in bowel frequency?*
d) *Other gastrointestinal disease?* e.g. mouth ulceration, anal fissuring, melaena, nausea and vomiting.

133

e) *Exacerbating factors?* e.g. cow's milk, fatty food.
f) *Urinary symptoms?*
g) *Family history?* e.g. RAP, migraine, anxiety disorders.
h) *Social circumstances?*

It is important to ask the parents whether they are concerned about any particular organic disease. Simple reassurance by the doctor may be all that is needed. It is also important to ask about any stresses the child may be under at home or at school.

A thorough physical examination is essential but rarely rewarding. Investigations will usually be of no diagnostic value and should only be performed if clinically indicated. At the first consultation I would only undertake urine microscopy and culture. Obvious features in the history and examination suggesting an organic cause will require investigation of the appropriate system.

Underlying anxieties may take many clinic visits before coming to light. Both child and parents must be taken seriously and criticism must not be levelled at parenting skills. Reassurance that there is nothing seriously wrong with the child, that the child requires no further invasive investigations and can lead a normal life is very therapeutic for both the child and the parents. Just as in adults, children can feel stress and anxiety and this can manifest itself as real symptoms, such as RAP. It is important that the child does not feel that no one takes the pain seriously. I would liaise with the school to avoid the child being repeatedly sent home. If there are problems in the home, social services involvement may be advantageous. Clinical psychologists may also have a role to play.

Reassurance that the abdominal pain should eventually settle down as the child grows up may not always be true, but in the vast majority of cases, it will be. Simple analgesia can be of benefit if it gives symptomatic relief, provided that it is not in excess. Long-term follow-up in the clinic is usually needed.

REFERENCE
Hyams J S, Hyams P E 1998 Recurrent abdominal pain and the biopsychosocial model of medical practice. J Pediatr 133: 473–478

FAILURE TO THRIVE

Q. What do you understand by the term 'failure to thrive'?

'Failure to thrive' is a descriptive term which suggests that a child has a rate of growth that does not meet the expected potential for a child of that age. I tend to use the term mainly for infancy and early childhood, when poor growth, particularly poor weight gain, is a common problem. It is a term that should be used with caution in front of families, as they might interpret the term 'failure' as a criticism of their care. 'Faltering growth' is an alternative term.

There are many causes of failure to thrive, which include nutritional problems and malabsorption, poor general health, and psychosocial problems.

Q. So, how would you identify these children?

General practitioners, community paediatricians, and health visitors have an important role in screening for growth. Plotting the weight and head circumference is routine for most infants at developmental checks and at the time of immunisations. Weight should be measured in the same state of dress on each occasion and should certainly be checked naked in infancy. When possible, the same set of weighing scales should be used on subsequent visits, because there may be a significant difference between scales. Length or height should be measured if there are concerns about growth.

Growth charts were updated in 1990. The new charts have centiles spreading at intervals of two-thirds of a standard deviation, from the 0.4th centile to the 99.8th centile. It is not possible to identify children who are failing to thrive from one measurement, but children who are below the 0.4th centile should be referred for assessment as they are markedly small and may have an underlying condition causing this.

The majority of children referred to the clinic are those who are 'falling' across the centile chart. It is important to remember that some infants have a good birth weight as a result of good maternal nutrition, whereas their 'programmed' size may be considerably smaller. These children will appear to fail to thrive in the first few weeks of life as they adjust to a centile which suits them. Both large and small babies will tend to 'regress to the mean' over the first few weeks of life, so it is important not to cause excessive anxiety when an infant of up to 6 weeks of age crosses a centile if that child is well and feeding appropriately.

Q. When would you investigate an infant who is failing to thrive?

Firstly, I would take a detailed history of the feeding pattern. It is often possible to identify simple reasons for poor weight gain, so avoiding the need for investigations. The amount of milk offered and taken should be ascertained. It might also be sensible to check how the mother is making up the milk in infants on formula feeds. For infants being weaned, I check that appropriate foods are being given, in particular whether gluten-free products are being used. The introduction of gluten-containing foods should alert you to the possibility of coeliac disease as a cause for the failure to thrive. I ask about the pattern of bowel habit, particularly whether the infant has loose, bulky, and offensive stools, suggestive of malabsorption.

It is important to check the height of both parents and preferably other siblings to see if the child is constitutionally small, as this may also prevent unnecessary investigations.

If it was clear from the history and examination that there is no obvious cause for the failure to thrive, I would undertake some baseline investigations. I would check a full blood count for signs of anaemia; renal and liver function tests to rule out renal and liver dysfunction; and thyroid function tests as hypothyroidism can cause failure to thrive. If the child has gluten in the diet I would check anti-endomysial antibodies to screen for coeliac disease. I always send a clean-catch specimen of urine, as urinary tract infection can cause few symptoms in the younger child. In a girl I would check chromosomes for Turner's syndrome, which may present as failure to grow, with few dysmorphic features. I would consider cystic fibrosis as a cause of malabsorption and arrange for a chest X-ray and sweat test to be performed if there was any doubt. If the child had a history of frequent infections I would check immunoglobulins as a screen for immune function.

If an infant continued to gain weight poorly I would arrange for admission to the ward as it is easier to assess feeding patterns by direct observation. If the child then gains weight I would be suspicious that the poor weight gain had been due to home circumstances and it would be important to arrange support at home for the family.

REFERENCE
Wright C M 2000 Identification and management of failure to thrive: a community perspective. Arch Dis Child 82: 5–9

MANAGEMENT OF GASTROENTERITIS

Q. Tell me how you would manage a child presenting to hospital with gastroenteritis.

I feel that there are two important issues in the management of this child:

1. What is the risk of dehydration occurring?
2. What is the severity of any dehydration already present?

The answer to the first question can be ascertained from the history and the second from the examination findings. Factors associated with an *increased risk of dehydration* include:

— age less than 12 months
— stool frequency >8/day
— vomiting >2/day
— underlying poor nutrition
— bottle-fed rather than breastfed infant

Features that are useful in assessing the *degree of dehydration* include the presence or absence of the following:

— decreased skin turgor
— dry oral mucosa
— sunken eyes
— altered level of consciousness

From my history and examination I would then have some assessment of whether the gastroenteritis was mild, moderate, or severe, although this is a somewhat arbitrary classification. Wherever possible, I would endeavour to use oral rehydration rather than intravenous fluids, bearing in mind that dehydration from gastroenteritis is associated with sodium and chloride losses and sometimes significant potassium depletion and acidosis. There are a number of oral rehydration solutions (ORS) available, each with different individual electrolyte concentrations. There is probably little, if any, advantage of one over the other. The fluid should be given 'little and often' to minimise the risk of vomiting — for example, 5 ml every 5 minutes rather than 60 ml once every hour.

Most children with gastroenteritis are thirsty and will want to drink but in those disinclined to, a nasogastric tube can be inserted and rehydration carried out in a similar way. Rather than attempting to rehydrate over a prolonged period (i.e. 24–48 hours, as for i.v. rehydration — see page 149), it is safe and effective to try and replace losses over 4 hours. If the child vomits or has ongoing stool losses, these volumes should be added to the calculated total fluid replacement. I would *consider* intravenous fluids in those children with shock, severe dehydration or persistent vomiting (see dehydration and rehydration).

Breastfeeding should continue throughout the rehydration process. For bottle-fed babies, milk should be reintroduced after 4 hours if the initial 4-hour rehydration process has been successful.

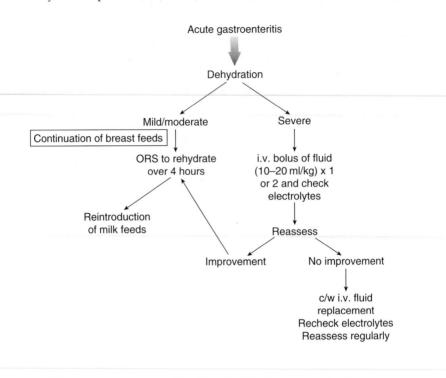

Q. Would you use any medication in the treatment of gastroenteritis?

The short answer to this question is, 'No'! I am not aware of any benefit in using antidiarrhoeal agents in the management of this very common condition. The question of whether or not to give antibiotics in acute gastroenteritis is not as straightforward. For the majority, the cause will be viral and obviously antibiotics are not indicated. For those with bacterial gastroenteritis, again, antibiotics may not be indicated. Exceptions to this are for *Salmonella* and *Shigella* gastroenteritis. For *Salmonella typhi* and *Salmonella paratyphi* infections I would treat with a course of oral ciprofloxacin and for *Shigella* I would use ampicillin or amoxicillin.

Q. OK, tell me what is found in oral rehydration solutions?

All commonly used oral rehydration solutions used in the UK (Dioralyte, Diocalm Junior, Rehidrat) contain sodium, potassium, chloride and glucose. The concentrations vary slightly, but are usually:

— sodium: 50–60 mmol/L
— potassium: 20–25 mmol/L

— chloride: 50–60 mmol/L
— glucose: 90–110 mmol/L

Some solutions also contain citrate and bicarbonate.

REFERENCES
Gastañaduy A S, Begue R E 1999. Acute gastroenteritis. Clin Pediatr 38: 1–12
Liebelt E L 1998 Clinical and laboratory evaluation and management of children with vomiting, diarrhea, and dehydration. Curr Opin Pediatr 10: 461–469
Murphy M S 1998 Guidelines for managing acute gastroenteritis based on a systematic review of published research. Arch Dis Child 79: 279–284

Gastroenterology and infection

PYREXIA OF UNKNOWN ORIGIN

Q. What is your approach to the child with a pyrexia of unknown origin?

Strictly speaking, the definition 'pyrexia of unknown origin' (PUO) is reserved for patients who have unexplained pyrexia for longer than 1 week. There is a long list of causes of PUO, but most cases in children are due to infection or autoimmune disease.

The *infectious causes* can be further divided into:

1. Bacterial (TB, SBE, abscesses, osteomyelitis)
2. Viral (EBV, CMV, HIV)
3. Protozoal (malaria, toxoplasmosis)
4. Fungal (histoplasmosis)

Important *autoimmune causes* include juvenile chronic arthritis (JCA), SLE, and inflammatory bowel disease. Neoplastic causes of PUO include leukaemia, lymphoma, and Wilms' tumour. Miscellaneous causes include Kawasaki disease, drug fevers, and factitious fevers.

It is important to take a thorough history, concentrating in particular on aspects such as foreign travel (malaria, brucellosis); the health of other family members (TB, HIV); and any pets and their health (psittacosis). Weight loss is important, as is the presence of sweats and rigors (which might indicate collection of pus). Sporting activities might point to possible diagnoses: potholers are at risk of histoplasmosis; water sports can give rise to leptospirosis. Parents do not normally volunteer such information, not knowing its importance, so such clues can only be detected by careful history-taking.

It is important to examine the child for subtle clinical signs, including a rash in JCA, a tick bite in typhus, or a rose spot in typhoid fever.

Q. How would you investigate such a child?

There is a long list of possible investigations but it is important to do these in a sensible order, guided by findings from the history and examination. *Initial investigations* should include FBC, as the type of white blood cells present will suggest whether there is infection of bacterial/viral or parasitic origin, and blood film, which would show abnormal cell types in leukaemia. It is usual to check the ESR or CRP, which are both valuable in tracking the progress of the disease process. Several sets of blood cultures should be taken, preferably when the child is febrile — particularly if bacterial endocarditis is suspected. A chest X-ray might show TB or lymphoma, when no clinical signs are present. Baseline serology is important, including viral titres and titres for atypical organisms such as *Rickettsia*, *Coxiella*, *Legionella*, *Mycoplasma* and *Toxoplasma*. It is worth asking the laboratory to store some serum for investigations which may be thought relevant later. Antistreptolysin O titre and autoantibody titres should be measured. If tuberculosis is suspected, I would perform a tuberculin test. Urine and stool should be cultured. Biopsy of any enlarged lymph node should be considered.

If the initial investigations show no cause for the fever, I would proceed to further *imaging investigations*. Depending on pointers from the history and examination, these might include abdominal ultrasound or CT for collections, white-cell scan, and barium studies. More invasive investigations may be indicated, depending on the history, examination, and initial investigations. These include lumbar puncture, rectal biopsy, endoscopy with biopsy, bone marrow aspiration, liver biopsy, or, rarely, diagnostic laparotomy.

It is usual practice to admit a child for investigation of fever of unknown origin. However, once the process of investigation has begun, it may be appropriate to allow the child to go home with a temperature chart, if she is not too unwell, while results are awaited.

Tip

- A rather general question like this is not too difficult and it is likely that the examiner will guide you towards a particular diagnosis that he wants to talk about.

INFLAMMATORY BOWEL DISEASE

Q. How would you manage a 13-year-old boy presenting with a one-month history of abdominal pain, weight loss and blood-stained diarrhoea?

I would be concerned that this boy has a form of inflammatory bowel disease. My initial assessment would include a detailed history of his abdominal pain and bowel habit. Lower abdominal pain, which is cramping in nature, is typical of ulcerative colitis but is not specific to that condition. The pain in Crohn's disease is often generalised but can be confined to the right lower quadrant in disease predominantly affecting the terminal ileum. The importance of asking about the bowel habit is that it gives an indication of the severity of the disease.

I would want to ask about symptoms of general ill health, particularly fever, fatigue, and poor appetite. Again, these are not specific to inflammatory bowel disease, but can be clues to anaemia and an inflammatory response. The presence of other symptoms, such as arthralgia and skin rashes, might help to confirm a diagnosis.

My examination would include an assessment of growth and, at this boy's age, pubertal status. Previous height and weight measurements would show whether his growth rate had faltered. I would look for clubbing and signs of clinical anaemia. Mouth ulcers can be present in both Crohn's disease and ulcerative colitis. Extreme tenderness or distension of the abdomen would indicate severe disease. A mass in the right iliac fossa may be present in Crohn's disease and may signify an abscess in the terminal ileum. A rectal examination might show perianal fistulae or tags. The boy might have swelling of the joints or restricted joint movement if he had described arthralgia, though it is unusual to see actual joint deformity.

Q. What investigations might be helpful?

It is important to exclude infectious causes of bloody diarrhoea, so I would send a stool sample for culture, looking for organisms such as *Salmonella*, *Shigella*, *Yersinia* and *E. coli*. If the boy had recently been treated with antibiotics I would also check for *Clostridium difficile* toxin. I would request a full blood count as children with inflammatory bowel disease may be anaemic with thrombocytosis and leucocytosis. Inflammatory markers, such as ESR and CRP, may be raised but the CRP is usually more noticeably raised in Crohn's disease than in ulcerative colitis. A low albumin secondary to gut protein loss is further evidence of inflammatory bowel disease.

Further investigations would depend on the clinical picture. For example, symptoms of predominantly colonic involvement in a child who is not currently toxic would lead me to arrange colonoscopy with biopsy. Rectal involvement with proximal extension might suggest ulcerative colitis, while rectal sparing with 'skip lesions' would be more in favour of a diagnosis of

Crohn's. Histology is not always definitive, but the presence of granulomata would suggest Crohn's. If there was significant upper abdominal pain or nausea, I would also arrange contrast-medium small-bowel studies with follow-through as this might show signs of small bowel wall thickening or ulceration.

Q. Fine. So what are you going to do to make this boy better?

Well, in the first instance I would want to give him symptomatic relief. If he had significant anaemia, I would give a *blood transfusion*. I would also offer *pain relief*. Aims of further treatment would be to reduce gastrointestinal and extraintestinal symptoms; to provide sufficient *nutrition* to allow growth; and to minimise disruption to ordinary life.

If investigations suggested the diagnosis of Crohn's disease, I would consider *enteral feeding* with either an elemental or semi-elemental diet. This means giving amino acids or protein hydrolysate. This has been shown to have a high rate of success in inducing both clinical and biochemical remission, with some evidence of histological remission. The diet preparations are not pleasant to take by mouth, so I would suggest placing a nasogastric tube for feeding. Other foods should not be given at the same time. The diet should be high in calories to make up for the weight loss and excess calories lost through malabsorption.

The *salicylate compounds* can be useful for colonic disease in both Crohn's disease and ulcerative colitis. The active moiety of the drug is 5-amino-salicylate but, as this is absorbed quickly in the small intestine, different formulations are used to allow it to reach the colon. Traditionally, sulfasalazine was used but this has a greater side-effect profile due to the sulfapyridine component, so mesalazine or olsalazine are being used more frequently.

Corticosteroids are also used in both forms of inflammatory bowel disease. These can be given intravenously in the severely unwell child, or orally in those able to tolerate them. Topical steroids in the form of enemas or foams can be useful in the child with rectal involvement. A course of high-dose steroids should continue for at least two weeks or until the bloody diarrhoea had settled. The dose would then be gradually reduced. If the child is steroid-dependent, an alternate-day regimen should be used in order to minimise the effects on growth. Sometimes it is necessary to use an alternative immunosuppressant, such as azathioprine, in a steroid-dependent child.

Q. With all these medical treatments, is there a role for surgery?

There are indications for surgery in both forms of inflammatory bowel disease. There may be a need for surgery to cope with acute complications, such as toxic megacolon, haemorrhage, or perforation. However, surgery is more commonly needed in intractable disease in ulcerative colitis, or when there is growth failure unresponsive to medical treatment. Occasionally, total colectomy is performed as prophylaxis against cancer, but this is done less commonly now as the reduction of inflammation by medical treatments is believed to reduce the incidence of cancer.

Surgical treatment in Crohn's disease is not curative but might be appropriate for localised disease where growth is slow or symptoms are resistant to medical treatment.

REFERENCE
Walker-Smith J A 1997 Therapy of Crohn's disease in childhood. Baillières Clin Gastroenterol 11(3): 593–610

HIV AND AIDS

Q. How do children become infected with HIV?

Mother-to-infant transmission (*vertical transmission*) of HIV accounts for 90% of AIDS in children. All new cases of HIV in children at present have resulted from vertical transmission. Transmission from an infected mother to her child can occur during pregnancy (in utero), at delivery (intrapartum) or during breastfeeding (postpartum). It is estimated that 25–40% of infections occur in utero and the remainder during labour and delivery. Transmission rates from infected mothers to children range from 16–20% in Europe and North America to 25–40% in Africa. The precise reason behind this large difference is still unknown, but the higher proportion of infected mothers who breast-feed their babies is thought to have a large influence. Breast milk from infected mothers contains HIV and the rate of infection in breastfed infants who are HIV- negative at birth is approximately 13%. The exact viral load required to cause infection is unknown, but it is thought that the majority of babies become infected in the first few months of breastfeeding. In the UK HIV-infected mothers are advised not to breastfeed; in Africa infected mothers are encouraged to breastfeed because of the greater risk of infant malnutrition. Delivery by caesarian section for infected women has been shown to reduce the transmission rate to approximately 10% and the use of antiretroviral drugs in pregnancy reduces the rate further, to approximately 5%.

Q. How is HIV infection diagnosed?

The method used for diagnosis of HIV in children depends on the age of the child. Up to 18 months of age, children of HIV-infected mothers may have IgG antibodies to HIV from transplacental transfer during pregnancy. In children over 18 months the presence of HIV IgG antibodies is diagnostic of HIV infection, although this must be confirmed by virological assay (HIV DNA PCR, HIV RNA PCR, or HIV culture). Children under 18 months must have the diagnosis made by virological assay. The most commonly used test is *HIV DNA PCR*, which is highly sensitive and specific (and the results are rapidly available). Children should have HIV DNA PCR performed at birth (avoid cord blood as this may be contaminated with maternal blood), at 1 month, and at 3 months. If children are positive at birth and also on subsequent tests, they are considered to have in-utero infection. Children who are negative at birth but who are positive on further tests are considered to have intrapartum infection. Other virology tests include HIV culture from peripheral lymphocytes (expensive and requires approximately 3 weeks) and HIV RNA PCR.

A number of other laboratory markers for HIV are used to provide additional evidence, although they are not diagnostic on their own. It is possible to detect antigen to the internal core protein of the virus (P24) by ELISA (enzyme-linked immunosorbent assay). T-helper lymphocytes with the CD4 cell-surface marker (CD4 cells) are reduced in HIV infection. In normal infants the CD4 count is initially very high, dropping to adult values by about 6 years of age. There may also be hypergammaglobulinaemia or, more rarely, hypogammaglobulinaemia.

Q. What about AIDS itself: how does the disease in children differ from that in adults?

About 20% of infants infected with HIV develop symptoms of AIDS in the first year of life. *Pneumocystis carinii* pneumonia (PCP) occurs at a much earlier stage in children than in adults. Most infants present with this and deteriorate very rapidly. The majority of children, however, do not develop symptoms until the age of 2 or 3 years.

Lymphoproliferative manifestations such as hepatosplenomegaly and parotid gland enlargement are common in children. Children may develop lymphoid interstitial pneumonitis (LIP), which is an infiltration of the lungs by lymphocytes almost never seen in adults. Central nervous system involvement in childhood AIDS is characterised by developmental delay or regression, and encephalopathy. However, unlike adult AIDS where superadded infections or CNS tumours occur, the deterioration in children is thought to be due to the virus itself. In general, neoplasms are much less common in childhood than in adult AIDS.

Q. What drugs are used in the treatment of HIV and AIDS?

There are now many antiretroviral drugs that are used in paediatric HIV infection and AIDS. The antiretroviral drugs fall into three groups: nucleoside reverse transcriptase inhibitors, non-nucleoside reverse transcriptase inhibitors and protease inhibitors.

1. *Nucleoside reverse transcriptase inhibitors (NRTI).* This class of drug inhibits the reverse transcriptase enzyme of the virus. The most commonly used drug in this group is zidovudine. Anaemia and neutropenia are the most common side-effects seen.
2. *Non-nucleoside reverse transcriptase inhibitors (NNRTI).* This class of drug binds directly to the enzymatic site of reverse transcriptase, resulting in inhibition. Drugs in this group include nevirapine — its major side-effects include hepatitis and skin rashes.
3. *Protease inhibitors.* This class of drug binds to, and inhibits, the viral protease. Drugs in this group include ritonavir and nelfinavir.

Recommendations for therapy vary from year to year. Current regimens usually consist of triple therapy, with two NRTIs and a protease inhibitor. With further research into HIV it is likely that new drugs will be developed.

The other common drug used in HIV infection is *cotrimoxazole*, which is used for prophylaxis against PCP.

Q. What vaccinations are given to children who are HIV positive?

Immunisation is an important part of the medical management of HIV infection. HIV-infected children should receive all the usual recommended vaccinations except for polio vaccine which should be given in the inactivated form instead of the oral (live) form. The other live vaccines (MMR) should be given, except for the BCG. Infants should also be given pneumococcal and influenza vaccinations.

REFERENCE
Bulterys M et al 1998 Mother-to-child transmission of HIV. Curr Opin Pediatr 10: 143–150

DEHYDRATION AND REHYDRATION

Q. How would you assess and treat dehydration in a child?

Assessment of dehydration is a clinical skill, that is used many times a day in general practice and in the casualty department of hospitals. The most important decisions are to the questions:

— Does this child need hospital admission for rehydration?
— Does this child need intravenous fluid replacement?

Should the answer to these questions be 'Yes', then the problem arises of 'How much' and 'What sort?'. Dehydration can be *classified* in two ways:

1. Tonicity: hypotonic
              isotonic
              hypertonic
2. Natraemic state: hyponatraemic — serum Na^+ <130 mmol/L
                     isonatraemic — serum Na^+ 130–150 mmol/L
                     hypernatraemic – serum Na^+ >150 mmol/L

The categories are not interchangeable.

Severity of dehydration, usually based on percentage body weight loss, may be mild (<5%), moderate (5–10%) or severe (>10%). The most accurate way to determine this is by finding out a recent body weight prior to the onset of the current illness and comparing this with admission weight. However, aspects of the history and examination must be elicited to confirm or determine your judgement. From the history, the frequency of micturition is very relevant: in mild dehydration urine output is essentially normal, in moderate dehydration output is reduced and concentrated; and with severe dehydration urine output is minimal and the last urine output may have occurred many hours previously. Of course, when there is a clinical picture of dehydration with inappropriate or excess urine output, diabetes mellitus, diabetes insipidus, and chronic renal failure must be excluded by appropriate investigation.

Clinical signs of dehydration include:

Mild (<5%)   Alert but restless child with normal BP and heart rate. Moist mucous membranes and normal skin elasticity

Moderate (5–10%)   Dry mucous membranes, sunken eyes and fontanelle (if appropriate), increased skin turgor

Severe (10%)   Drowsy, irritable child with cool peripheries, rapid and feeble pulses. Very sunken eyes and markedly increased skin turgor. Coma and unrecordable BP in more severe cases

My *initial investigation and management* for a child requiring hospital admission and intravenous rehydration therapy would involve:

1. Weighing the child
2. I.V. access: FBC + haematocrit, U & Es + osmolality, glucose
3. I.V. HAS/0.9% normal saline, 20 ml/kg over 30 minutes if shocked
4. Strict input and output measurement
5. Measurement of urine osmolality and electrolytes if severe, especially if there is polyuria in the presence of dehydration

Intravenous *fluid volumes required* must be calculated, taking into account maintenance fluids and correction of the deficit, +/− replacement of ongoing losses:

— *Maintenance fluids* (per hour)
   4 ml/kg for the 1st 10 kg body weight
   2 ml/kg for the next 10 kg body weight
   1 ml/kg for every kg body weight above 20 kg
— *Deficit fluids*
   % dehydration × body weight × 10 = total fluid deficit (ml)

The total fluid deficit is divided into 24 to 48 equal aliquots (depending on whether rehydration is to be over 24 or 48 hours) and added to the hourly maintenance fluids
— *Replacement fluids*, i.e. urine, stool, vomitus, blood. Fluid should be replaced with like, usually 0.45% or 0.9% N/saline + KCl, in equal volume to the previous 1–4 hours' losses, depending on the severity of dehydration

a) *Hypotonic dehydration.* I would use either 0.45% or 0.9% N/Saline (80 mmol/L and 156 mmol/L respectively) and rehydrate over 24 hours.
   Calculation of sodium deficit for a child of 20 kg with a serum sodium of 115 mmol/L and 10% (2000 ml) dehydration:
   Deficit $= ((135–115) \times \text{weight} \times 0.6 \text{ (i.e. ECF*)}) + (\text{fluid deficit} \times 115)$
   $= (20 \times 20 \times 0.6) + (2 \times 115)$
   $= 470 \text{ mmol Na}^+$
   *as majority of Na^+ is in ECF
   The child with severe hypotonic dehydration will have a metabolic acidosis but I would rarely, if ever, correct this with an infusion of sodium bicarbonate. Electrolyte and fluid correction will bring up the serum pH in a much more physiological manner.
b) *Isotonic dehydration.* Again, correction over 24 hours is acceptable and I would use 0.45% saline/2.5% dextrose after initial resuscitation fluids, provided the serum glucose was adequate.
c) *Hypertonic dehydration.* I would correct this more slowly, taking 48 hours at least, to reduce the risk of cerebral oedema and possible seizures. Assessment of dehydration is difficult because the usual clinical signs of severe dehydration may be lacking, i.e. increase in skin turgor, sunken fontanelle. After initial resuscitation I would use either 0.45% N/Saline or 0.18% N/Saline (=32 mmol/L Na^+), aiming to bring the serum sodium down by no more than 5 mmol per 24 hours.

In all three types of dehydration, the addition of KCL to the rehydration fluids is titrated against serum K^+ measurement and urine output.

Gastroenterology and infection

Q. What are the causes of polyuria?

Polyuria can be defined as a urine output of greater than 4 ml/kg/hour for longer than 2 consecutive hours. I have found that it is not an infrequent reason for referral to the clinic by GPs, as a result of parental anxiety. In almost all cases, polyuria is simply a result of polydipsia in a well child who enjoys drinking (or is given a drink as a pacifier!). Taking a history, examining the child, and dipsticking the urine is often all that is necessary to exclude disease. However, there are a number of conditions in which polyuria is a prominent feature. These include:

— water overload: iatrogenic or psychogenic polydipsia
— diabetes insipidus
— renal tubular acidosis
— hypercalcaemia
— recovery phase of acute renal failure
— osmotic diuresis, especially hyperglycaemia
— diuretics and other drug ingestion
— cerebral salt wasting

Q. Give me some other formulae that may be used when there are fluid and electrolyte problems.

I have found the following useful in the more complicated cases of dehydration:

1. *Insensible water loss*:
    newborn — 25 ml/kg/day
    child — 15 ml/kg/day
    adult — 250 ml/m²/day

2. *Surface area* (if height not known):
    $$\text{Surface area (m}^2) = \frac{(\text{weight} \times 4) + 7}{\text{weight} + 90}$$

3. *Fractional sodium excretion*:

    $$FE_{Na} = \frac{\text{urine Na}^+}{\text{urine creatinine}} \times \frac{\text{plasma creatinine}}{\text{Plasma Na}^+}$$

    Normal is < 1%. It is high with excess sodium intake, water overload, renal salt wasting disorders and with diuretics.

4. *Osmolality*:
    Osmolality (mosmol/kg) = $1.86 \times (\text{Na}^+ + \text{K}^+) + \text{gluc} + \text{creat} + 10$
    If measured osmolality is > 5 mosomol/kg greater than calculated, there is another solute present e.g. ethanol, ethylene glycol.

5. *Anion gap*:
    Anion gap (meq/L) = $\text{Na}^+ + \text{K}^+ - \text{Cl}^- - \text{HCO}_3$
    The anion gap is the unmeasured anions, e.g. lactate, ketones, drugs, organic acids.

Tip

● Some of these formulae are difficult to remember. In reality, the safest approach to intravenous rehydration is: do it slowly; use isotonic fluids (0.45% saline + 2.5% dextrose +/− KCl); and recheck the serum electrolytes regularly to ensure things are going in the right direction (but not too quickly). For younger children a higher concentration of dextrose may, of course, be necessary.

VOMITING

Q. As the paediatric registrar on call, you are called to the postnatal ward by your SHO to review a 2-day-old baby with severe vomiting who looks unwell. Outline your differential diagnosis.

This is a common problem and must be investigated thoroughly, as the aetiology is often serious. Salient features of the history include:

1. Antenatal history — consanguinity, polyhydramnios, ultrasound scans, evidence of maternal sepsis.
2. Feeding — bottle, breast, frequency, volume.
3. Vomitus — bile, blood, milk.
4. Meconium — ? passed.

I would make a full clinical examination of the infant, looking specifically for evidence of sepsis and abdominal distension and checking for a patent anus. My differential diagnosis at this stage would be: sepsis, intestinal obstruction, or an inborn error of metabolism. The most common cause is *intestinal obstruction*, so my initial investigations would include FBC, U&E, chest X-ray, and abdominal X-ray. I would stop all feeds, pass a nasogastric tube, and give intravenous fluids, including replacement of nasogastric fluid draining. If there was clear evidence of obstruction on the AXR I would ask for a surgical opinion. If I felt that the child was *septic* I would perform a full septic screen, including lumbar puncture, CXR, AXR, blood cultures and suprapubic aspiration of urine. I would then start intravenous fluids and prescribe ampicillin and gentamicin. To exclude *a metabolic* problem I would perform a capillary pH, serum ammonia, serum glucose and send blood for amino acids and organic acids.

Q. You are referred a 5-month-old in outpatients with recurrent vomiting. What are you going to do?

This is an extremely common referral to paediatric outpatients. In over 90% of cases the diagnosis will be *gastro-oesophageal reflux* (GOR), but it is essential to exclude pathological causes by means of thorough history-taking, examination, and investigation as indicated. Salient features of the history include:

1. Timing of the vomiting — i.e. related or unrelated to feeds. More relevant if *not* related to feeds.
2. Nature of the vomiting — i.e. possetting or vomiting, effortless, projectile.
3. Nature of the vomitus — i.e. bile-stained, bloodstained, curdled milk.
4. Onset of the vomiting — after 6 weeks of age it is unlikely to be GOR.
5. Is the infant thriving? — simple GOR does not cause failure to thrive.
6. Associated features — diarrhoea, steatorrhoea, bloody stools, cough.

The answers to these questions would direct me to the most likely aetiology.

I would not undertake any further investigations (except urine culture) unless I suspected a pathological aetiology or the child was failing to thrive. I would give advice that might minimise GOR, such as: elevation of the head of the cot; not nursing the baby in a sitting position after feeds (as this is the worst anti-reflux position); and thickening of the feeds with carobel (1 scoop to 100 ml of milk and enlarge the aperture of the teat). Gaviscon, ranitidine and omeprazole can be given on a trial basis, although I am not aware of any controlled studies demonstrating their benefit in simple GOR.

The natural history of GOR is that the vomiting settles down by 18 months of age as the child adopts a more upright posture, although a significant proportion will settle down much earlier. I would review the infant in the outpatient department 1 month after starting treatment to assess for symptomatic improvement and appropriate weight gain.

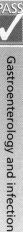

DIARRHOEA

Q. You are called to casualty to see a 1-year-old boy with a four-day history of diarrhoea. Outline your management.

Diarrhoea is one of the most common reasons for children to be brought to a doctor and in the majority of cases they can be managed at home. Infective agents causing diarrhoea can be divided into *viral* (rotavirus, astrovirus, calicivirus, and Norwalk virus), *bacterial* (*Salmonella, Shigella, Campylobacter* and *E.coli*) and *parasitic* (*Giardia lamblia, Entamoeba histolytica*).

Important factors that I would want to elicit in the *history* include the duration (number of days); frequency (times per day), nature (?watery, ?offensive, colour, froth, blood, mucus); and timing (relation to meals) of diarrhoea and whether there has been any associated vomiting. I would establish how much fluid the child is managing to drink and the number of wet nappies over the last 24 hours. It is useful to know whether any other children at home or at nursery have diarrhoea and whether there has been any recent foreign travel.

It is important to undertake a full *examination* of the child. An assessment of the child's hydration, specifically skin turgor, anterior fontanelle tension, urine output, mental status, mucous membrane hydration, blood pressure, and peripheral perfusion, is essential. It is worthwhile weighing the patient, as the parents may know a recent weight for comparison.

Most children attending casualty require no investigation and, providing the child is managing oral fluids and passing urine, simple reassurance and advice is all that is necessary. Oral rehydration solutions (ORS) can be prescribed for the parents to use at home. Children not managing oral fluids or who are severely dehydrated will require admission to hospital. These children will require U&E (to give further evidence of the degree of dehydration and to allow provision of appropriate rehydration fluids), stool culture and possibly intravenous fluids.

Q. You are asked to see a 3-year-old in outpatients who has been referred by the GP with chronic diarrhoea. Outline how you would proceed.

Chronic diarrhoea is defined as the passage of loose stools for more than 2 weeks and is a common referral to paediatric outpatients. There are many causes and a thorough history and examination, together with some simple investigations, will often yield the diagnosis and spare children unnecessary invasive procedures. The age of the child at presentation is important as many conditions tend to be age-specific. The most common conditions causing chronic diarrhoea in infants are toddler's diarrhoea, secondary disaccharidase deficiency, and cow's milk protein intolerance.

Toddler's diarrhoea is seen in children aged between 6 months and 3 years. The child is generally well and the diarrhoea is classically described as 'peas and carrots diarrhoea', containing visible undigested food. Examination will reveal a normal child with normal weight and height. The aetiology of this condition is poorly understood, although failure to chew food adequately and rapid gastrointestinal transit time have been implicated. These children require no further investigation other than stool culture to exclude covert infection such as giardiasis. There is no specific treatment, although some children improve when the fat content of the diet is increased by Calogen, which reduces the gut transit time.

Secondary disaccharidase deficiency (usually lactase) is commonly precipitated by an attack of gastroenteritis. Temporary withdrawal of milk (and, if necessary, other carbohydrate-containing foods from the diet) may improve the symptoms.

Cow's milk protein intolerance is a rare cause of diarrhoea in infants and can sometimes resemble toddler's diarrhoea, although food particles are absent from the stools. Tests for this condition are complicated and, therefore, if the diagnosis is suspected milk is empirically withdrawn from the diet and improvement in symptoms usually establishes the diagnosis clinically. Small amounts of milk accidentally ingested thereafter may induce an acute reaction with vomiting, diarrhoea, urticaria, and bronchospasm. Occasionally, chronic exposure may cause severe failure to thrive, rectal bleeding, and hepatosplenomegaly, caused by an immunological reaction to milk protein.

Three conditions that may present at any age in childhood are giardiasis, coeliac disease, and cystic fibrosis. These conditions often show features of malabsorption so I would make a specific enquiry about the passage of offensive, pale, fatty stools which float and may be difficult to flush away.

Giardiasis is caused by the flagellate protozoan, *Giardia lamblia*, which primarily affects the duodenum and upper jejunum. It produces offensive fatty motions due to secondary disaccharidase deficiency. The trophozoite of *Giardia* may be seen on stool microscopy. Duodenal aspiration or examination of a jejunal biopsy (which may show villous atrophy as well as parasitic cysts) is necessary in a few children to establish the diagnosis. The treatment of choice is metronidazole.

A child with *coeliac disease* usually has symptoms dating from the introduction of gluten-containing foods and will appear miserable, with a poor appetite and abdominal distension. It typically presents at 5–7 months but can present at any age.

A child with *cystic fibrosis* may have a history of persistent cough, recurrent pneumonia or nasal polyposis.

I would consider *inflammatory bowel disease* as a possible cause if there was a history of bloody or mucous diarrhoea, significant abdominal pain, oral signs (including ulceration), or anal disease.

Less common causes of chronic diarrhoea include *laxative abuse*, *pseudomembranous colitis*, *thyrotoxicosis* and *factitious illness*.

Q. OK, I'll stop you there. How would you investigate this patient?

This would depend on the age of the patient; the nature of the stools; the presence of any significant systemic symptoms; the presence of any abnormal signs; and the growth chart. It would be reasonable in many cases, as an *initial assessment*, to arrange: stool examination (and, where appropriate, multiple samples and a laxative screen); a full blood count to look for anaemia; ESR, as an inflammatory marker; U&E; serum albumin, which is reduced in malabsorptive conditions; and thyroid function tests to exclude thyrotoxicosis.

Other investigations to consider would be small-bowel aspiration and/or biopsy for detection of the flattened villi associated with coeliac disease; sigmoidoscopy with biopsy for inflammatory bowel disease; and a sweat test to exclude cystic fibrosis. In addition, in cases where the diagnosis is uncertain, I would use admission of the child to hospital as an investigation in its own right, to witness stool nature and frequency and to assess abnormal behaviour and possible laxative abuse.

Tip

● This may seem an easy question but many examiners will use it as an introduction to talk about other topics, such as the different features of dehydration or the salt and sugar composition of different types of oral rehydration solutions, both of which you should know.

Endocrinology, growth, and renal medicine

6

GROWTH HORMONE REPLACEMENT

Q. In what conditions would you use growth hormone?

Up until the mid-1980s growth hormone (GH) was obtained from the pituitary glands of cadavers. As a result, supplies were limited (fortunately, because of the transmission of Creutzfeld-Jakob disease). Since then recombinant growth hormone production has given us the opportunity to treat as many children as require it, bearing in mind the cost implications of growth hormone therapy. There are a significant number of conditions in which growth hormone has been used:

— growth hormone deficiency
— Turner's syndrome
— Down's syndrome
— Russell-Silver syndrome
— constitutional delay of growth and puberty (see page 159)
— chronic renal failure
— intrauterine growth retardation
— Prader-Willi syndrome
— idiopathic short stature

Of these conditions, few would argue against its use in GH deficiency. The younger the patient and the more severe the GH deficiency, the better the anticipated response to treatment.

The arguments for its use in conditions such as Turner's syndrome, Russell-Silver syndrome, Down's syndrome, chronic renal failure, etc. are less straightforward.

In children with *idiopathic short stature* (ISS), the situation is even less clear: proponents rely on the argument that it is effective in improving height, which in turn generates significant psychosocial benefit. There is certainly evidence of an increase in growth velocity in most children with GH therapy. However, long-term controlled studies looking at final adult height attained are lacking. The detractors of GH replacement in idiopathic short stature have persuasive arguments against its use. Height is normally distributed and so, by definition, 2 out of every 100 'normal' children will be below the 2nd centile. Why should a small normal child be a suitable candidate for a very expensive therapy with potential side-effects? I have seen this indication for GH therapy described as 'cosmetic endocrinology' by those opposed to its use. If society deems that being short is wrong and warrants treatment, the detractors would argue that it is society that is wrong, not the small child. I have certainly seen parents of a small child in the clinic pushing for GH replacement based on their belief in the perceived benefit of being tall.

Q. If *you* were the consultant sitting in the clinic seeing a child whose parents were pushing for GH replacement, would you recommend its use?

Based on the current evidence, which suggests that GH accelerates not only growth velocity, but also skeletal maturation, so resulting in a mean final height just above that predicted without GH, I would not recommend its routine use in ISS.

Tip

● If you get pushed 'off the fence' by the examiner, try to fall into the garden, where the evidence-based medicine family live! Of course there is always the easy answer of 'I would seek the advice of my nearest tertiary hospital paediatric endocrinologist!'

REFERENCES

Guyda H J 1999 Four decades of growth hormone therapy for short children: what have we achieved? J Clin Endocrinol Metab 84: 4307–4316

Voss L D, Saenger P 2000 Growth hormone therapy for the short normal child: who needs it and who wants it? J Pediatr 136: 103–110

SHORT STATURE AND CONSTITUTIONAL DELAY IN GROWTH AND PUBERTY

Q. Tell me how you would investigate a child with short stature.

The causes of short stature can be divided into five main categories:

1. Constitutional delay of growth and puberty (CDGP)
2. Familial short stature
3. Chronic disease
4. Genetic/chromosomal abnormalities
5. Endocrinopathies

The management is different for each category, so I would assess the child by means of a good history and examination and a few basic investigations to establish the diagnosis.

CDGP

This is defined as a delay of growth in an otherwise healthy child, with a standing height below the expected for chronological age, but not for bone age. It should be a diagnosis of exclusion and does not usually require treatment because final adult height will be within the normal range. Asking the parents when *they* went through puberty may demonstrate a familial tendency to CDGP. Calculating bone age from a wrist X-ray (conventionally the left) will reassure the child that they will catch up with their peers in time.

Familial short stature

Again, because this is a nonpathological condition, it should be a diagnosis of exclusion. A child's *expected final height* can be calculated using the following formulae:

For a girl, expected height $= \dfrac{(\text{father's height} - 12\ \text{cm}) + \text{mother's height}}{2}$

For a boy, expected height $= \dfrac{\text{father's height} + (\text{mother's height} + 12\ \text{cm})}{2}$

However, this can only be a rough guide to final height and caution must be taken when predicting final height with a child and parents — 'You said I would be 5 feet and 4 inches tall, and I am only 5 feet and 3 inches!'

Chronic illness, chromosomal and endocrine abnormalities

This really speaks for itself. The history and examination will hopefully yield useful clues to the cause for this child's short stature. Two diagnoses that are particularly important to think about are *Turner's syndrome* and *acquired hypothyroidism*. I have worked in one hospital where chromosomes (in the girls) and thyroid function were tested in all children referred for short stature, but this blanket policy is not adopted in other centres. The problem with making these two diagnoses is that the clinical signs and symptoms can be very subtle.

Whatever the suspected cause of short stature, I would usually see the child in the clinic again in 6 months, or sooner if specific pathologies were considered likely. At this second consultation it is possible to calculate the child's growth velocity (or height gain, as endocrinologists now like to call it) for the period of time between consultations. If the child is not falling across the centiles (or, in the good old days, growing at least 5 cm/year!) and I had no concerns arising from the history, examination or initial investigations, I would not see them again. Falling through the centiles (a growth velocity/height gain below 5 cm a year) should be taken seriously and would require further follow-up and possible investigation.

Q. Tell me a little bit more about CDGP.

Constitutional delay of growth and puberty (CDGP) is defined as delay of growth and puberty in otherwise healthy adolescents, with relatively reduced stature for chronological age, but generally appropriate for bone age. Since growth potential is related to the degree of epiphyseal maturation, the delay in bone age means that the child will have a final stature within the normal range for the parental heights.

It tends to affect more boys than girls. This is probably due to the difference in sensitivity to gonadotrophin-releasing hormone between the sexes. Girls produce gonadotrophins in response to small amounts of gonadotrophin-releasing hormone, which explains why precocious puberty is more common in girls. Boys are much less sensitive to gonadotrophin-releasing hormone and therefore puberty normally occurs later in adolescence. In CDGP the gonadotrophin-releasing hormone stimulation of gonadotrophin release occurs even later.

CDGP is a common cause of growth delay and is probably just an extreme of the normal range of growth patterns. Extensive investigation is unnecessary and the biochemical results may be misleading. The diagnosis should be made on anthropometric evidence, with the child demonstrating relatively short spinal length compared to leg length.

Q. Should these children be treated?

Although CDGP seems to be a physiological variant of normal, it can cause enormous anxiety for the affected individual. Peer-group pressure is very influential during puberty and comparison with others can cause significant distress. Boys are more commonly affected (because it is not such a problem for a girl to be small and they rarely present to their doctor) and tend to suffer more due to social pressures. The boy may be bullied and his behaviour may become deviant, leading to truancy, shoplifting, vandalism, etc. Treatment may therefore allow the boy to keep pace with his peers and avoid these social disadvantages. Interestingly, it has been shown that, although distressed during adolescence, most patients do not continue to have low self-esteem in adult life.

Adults who have had untreated CDGP do, however, seem to be at higher risk of later osteoporosis and persistent skeletal disproportion, i.e. they have a relatively short spine compared to leg length. For these reasons, it would seem sensible to treat these adolescents if a safe and effective treatment is available and if they are significantly distressed.

Q. OK, what treatments are available?

Treatments used in CDGP are based on the normal physiology of growth, which requires both growth hormone and sex steroids: changes in growth velocity are secondary to changes in the pulse amplitude of growth hormone, which is mainly secreted at night; sex steroids temporarily increase growth hormone secretion.

Treatment options include:

1. *Anabolic steroids*, e.g. oxandralone. These work by increasing growth hormone secretion. A low-dose daily regimen will induce a growth spurt, which continues once the steroids are stopped. They induce normal advancement in secondary sexual characteristics and have been shown to double the height-gain velocity. Previously they were used in high doses, but this caused inappropriate advancement of bone age and therefore a lower than predicted final height. This is not a problem at low dosage. Final height is not improved, but accelerated.
2. *Testosterone*. This induces the appearance of secondary sexual characteristics, but the levels of hormone tend to fluctuate, whether given orally or by deep i.m. depot injection. Testosterone should be given for a period of 3 months to allow a sustained growth spurt. (*Oestrogen* will have the same effect in girls.) *Human chorionic gonadotrophin* is a more physiological method of increasing sex hormones, but has to be given by injection three times a week to produce sustained levels. Sex steroids can be used when inadequate sexual development is the main complaint.
3. *Growth hormone*. This has been used mainly in growth-hormone deficient children. It has, however, been shown to increase height-gain velocity in boys with constitutional delay if given in high doses over a long period of time.

Tips

● The subject of short stature lends itself well to a 'hunt the diagnosis' type of question, for example, '*I have got this boy sitting in the clinic who complains that he is shorter than his school friends. Ask me some questions to sort out what the problem could be*'. It would still be reasonable to open with a broad introduction to the diagnostic categories and then to tailor your questioning to the likely group the child falls into.

● Do not forget the parent-held record book, which may give very useful clues as to the likely diagnosis. Look at the centile charts in this to see if the problem is short-or long-standing.

RECENT DEVELOPMENTS IN DIABETES

Q. Can you tell us of any recent developments in the care of children with diabetes mellitus?

There has been a change of emphasis in the management of children with diabetes mellitus since the publication of the Diabetes Control and Complications Trial in 1993. It had always been suspected that blood sugar control was related to the long-term complications of diabetes, but this trial showed conclusively that it is possible to delay the onset of microvascular complications such as retinopathy, neuropathy and nephropathy by using intensive insulin therapy regimens in a selected population of people with insulin-dependent diabetes mellitus.

It is not certain whether these results can be directly applied to children because the trial only included children over the age of 13 years. It was also conducted in highly motivated people who had more support during the trial period than is currently practical for long-term management in a clinic situation with limited resources. There were considerable increases in the incidence of hypoglycaemia and of weight gain, particularly in the adolescent age group, which both cause anxiety in many children and their families. Most paediatricians accept the need for an improvement in blood-sugar control in children, but are wary of increasing the incidence of hypoglycaemia, particularly in young children where neuroglycopenia might affect development and intelligence.

More units are using *multiple insulin injections* in an effort to be more flexible and therefore improve compliance, as well as to aim for a more physiological insulin regime. However, this depends on the patient being sufficiently motivated to test blood sugar and alter insulin doses regularly.

New insulins are being developed which mimic the action of intrinsic insulin more closely. These *insulin analogues* are designed to be absorbed quickly and can be injected immediately before a meal, which means that the peak plasma insulin level is more likely to correspond with the peak glucose level after a meal. It also reduces the chances of hypoglycaemia late after a meal. The insulin analogues are currently licensed for use in the older child, but might also prove to be very useful in toddlers where the threat of refusal to eat causes anxiety about hypoglycaemia once an insulin injection has been given.

It is recognised that improvement in blood glucose control is not simply a matter of changing insulin dosage. Diabetes services also need to ensure that the child and family are well informed about diabetes and receive good dietary advice.

REFERENCE
The diabetes control and complications trial research group 1999. The effect of intensive treatment of diabetes on the development and progression of long-term complications in insulin-dependent diabetes mellitus. N Engl J Med 329: 977–986

URINARY TRACT INFECTION

Q. How would you diagnose urinary tract infections in children?

Confirmed urinary tract infections (UTI) occur in approximately 3% of girls and 1% of boys during childhood. Diagnosis of a urinary tract infection requires a pure culture of $>10^5$ organisms/ml of a single organism and pyuria of at least 50×10^9/L; the presence of *any* organisms in a suprapubic aspirate is significant. *Collection of urine* in children is difficult and the method used is age-dependent.

1. *Children under 1 year of age*
   Suprapubic aspiration (SPA) is the gold standard — a growth of any organism is a positive result. Bag urine/'clean catch' methods are more commonly performed but are less satisfactory as they are often contaminated.
2. *Children aged 1–3 years*
   Clean-catch urine and mid-stream urine (MSU) are best although bag urines are often sent.
3. *Children over 3 years old*
   MSU is the most appropriate method.

   In all cases, except for SPA, I would want two specimens before starting antibiotics.

Q. What further investigations would you perform in a child with a proven UTI?

Again, the investigations would depend on the age of the child.

1. *Children under 2 years old*
   These children should have a renal ultrasound scan during their hospital stay, followed by a micturating cystourethrogram (MCUG) and DMSA scan 6–8 weeks later. It is important to leave this period of time to allow any inflammation to settle as this will influence the results. It is important to ensure that the child remains on prophylactic antibiotics until the investigations are completed.
2. *Children aged 2–5 years*
   These children should have a renal ultrasound and DMSA scan. If the child has recurrent UTIs, a family history of vesicoureteric reflux (VUR), or an abnormal DMSA scan, then a MCUG should be performed. Some of these children may need to stay on long-term prophylactic antibiotics.
3. *Children over 5 years old*
   These children should have a renal ultrasound scan unless other investigations are indicated.

Q. What is the difference between a DMSA scan and a DTPA scan?

A *DMSA Scan* (^{99m}Tc dimercaptosuccinic acid scintigraphy) is the gold standard for investigation of renal scars. DMSA is selectively taken up by the renal tubules and gamma radiation is emitted — renal scars show up as parenchymal filling defects on the scan. It cannot differentiate between acute and chronic scarring however.

A *DTPA Scan* (^{99m}Tc diethylenetriamine pentaacetic acid scan) is a *functional* test of the renal tract and is useful in differentiating between simple dilatation (i.e. megaureter) and obstructive dilatation (i.e. vesicoureteric junction or pelviureteric junction obstruction).

REFERENCES

Coward R J M 1999 An evidence-based appraisal of the investigation of childhood urinary tract infections. Curr Paediatr 9: 215–221

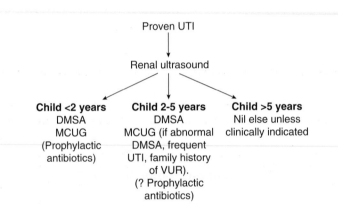

PRECOCIOUS PUBERTY

Q. How would you define precocious puberty?

Precocious puberty is the development of pubertal signs before the age of 8 years in a girl, and before the age of 9 years in a boy. Puberty is said to be 'central' if puberty is triggered by gonadotrophin-releasing hormone (GnRH), or 'GnRH-independent' if the hypothalamus is not activated.

Q. Why is there a difference between the sexes in age of onset of puberty?

Puberty starts when pulsatile release of GnRH from the hypothalamus increases, which triggers the release of follicle-stimulating hormone and luteinising hormone from the pituitary gland. These in turn activate gonadal function. The ovaries are more sensitive to gonadotrophin stimulation than the testes, so early puberty is more common in girls.

Q. How would you investigate precocious puberty in a boy?

While precocious puberty is relatively common in girls, it is uncommon in boys and there is more likely to be an identifiable cause. I would start by taking a detailed history of the *pattern of development*, asking, for example, whether there was change in the penis and testes prior to pubic hair development, as would be normal in male development, or whether pubic hair developed without a corresponding increase in testicular volume, as might happen in *congenital adrenal hyperplasia*. I would ask whether the boy has been having any headaches or vomiting suggestive of raised intracranial pressure, as *central nervous system tumours* are an important cause of precocious puberty in boys. I would ask about a history of encephalitis, epilepsy, severe head injury, or cranial irradiation as these may all cause precocious puberty.

On examination, I would check the boy's height and weight centiles in relation to the mid-parental height. I would expect the boy to be tall for family height in precocious puberty. I would specifically look for birthmarks as the *McCune-Albright syndrome* is associated with precocious puberty in both sexes. I would examine for signs of puberty, particularly testicular volume. If the testes are an appropriate size for the stage of puberty, it would suggest *central precocious puberty*. If one testis is significantly larger than the other, it might suggest a *hormone-producing testicular tumour*. If both testes are small, it suggests that the androgens have come from an alternative source, such as the adrenal glands.

I would check the boy's bone age and expect it to be advanced. Baseline hormonal levels may not be helpful, but I would arrange for a GnRH stimulation test, which would differentiate GnRH-dependent from GnRH-independent causes of precocious puberty. I would also check 17-hydroxy progesterone levels if suspicious of congenital adrenal hyperplasia and β-human chorionic gonadotrophin levels as these might be raised by liver tumours causing precocious puberty. I would want to do a head scan on all boys with unexplained precocious puberty, preferably an MRI scan as this is better at picking up small hamartomas in the hypothalamus.

Q. You mentioned McCune-Albright syndrome. What is the mechanism of precocious puberty in these children?

Normally, gonadotrophins bind to a receptor on the cell surface of the gonads which signals, via G proteins, the activation of an enzyme cascade producing cyclic AMP which then leads to the production of testosterone. In McCune-Albright syndrome, it is thought that there is a mutation leading to greater activation of the stimulatory G protein, causing excessive cyclic AMP resulting in excessive oestrogen or testosterone production.

RENAL FAILURE

Q. A 10-year-old boy is referred with lethargy, poor appetite, and hypertension. What would you do?

The hypertension suggests that the boy has renal failure and a history might help to establish whether this is *acute* or *chronic*. I would want to know how long the boy had been unwell and whether he had noticed any change in the amount of urine he passed. I would enquire about haematuria, suggestive of an acute nephritis, and frothy urine, suggestive of the proteinuria associated with nephrotic syndrome. I would ask whether he had recently had a sore throat, which might suggest post-streptococcal infection, or diarrhoea, which might suggest haemolytic uraemic syndrome. I would also enquire about a history of previous urinary tract infections or a family history of renal problems, for example polycystic renal disease.

My examination would include rechecking his *blood pressure*, looking for *anaemia* and generalised *oedema*, and checking for palpable kidneys. I would also examine his fundi, as signs of *retinopathy* would suggest a prolonged history of hypertension. Height and weight measurements are useful, as *short stature* would suggest chronic renal failure.

My initial investigations would include *urea, creatinine* and *electrolytes*, including calcium and phosphate. I would also check his *full blood count*, looking for normocytic, normochromic anaemia, and a blood film, looking for a haemolytic picture. I would *dipstick a urine sample*, checking for haematuria and proteinuria, then send it for microscopy to look for cell casts and culture. I would arrange for an urgent *renal ultrasound*, as this would give valuable information about the size and texture of the kidneys, as well as excluding cysts. If the kidneys are swollen, this might suggest acute inflammation, whereas shrunken kidneys are more likely to be a sign of chronic inflammation, as in reflux nephropathy for example. Further investigations would depend on the results of these preliminary tests.

Q. Fine. It turns out that the boy has chronic renal failure related to a history of recurrent urinary tract infections. How would you manage him?

This will depend firstly on whether there are any *indications for immediate dialysis*, such as uncontrolled hyperkalaemia, or fluid overload causing pulmonary oedema. Assuming that this is not the case, I would admit the boy to hospital and concentrate on the correction of hypertension, nutritional needs, and anaemia.

The *hypertension* is likely to be due to the underlying renal pathology, but may also be related to fluid overload. Treatment should be initiated as soon as possible, as control of hypertension might improve the glomerular filtration rate. Treatment sublingually with nifedipine or an oral beta-blocker is reasonable, as long as there is no history of asthma. If the blood pressure was high enough to cause encephalopathy, I would use either intravenous labetolol or sodium nitroprusside, preferably while monitoring arterial blood pressure. I would aim to reduce the blood pressure slowly, as a rapid reduction might cause sudden changes in cerebral perfusion pressure, leading to ischaemia.

Poor *nutrition* is often a problem in chronic renal failure and I would ask a dietician to be involved in further management. The child will need a high-calorie diet that is low in added salts. He may be able to eat a normal diet with added calorie supplements, but if weight gain is poor, nasogastric feeds should be considered.

Poor nutrition may be a contributary factor in the *anaemia* of chronic renal failure, which is compounded by reduced erythropoietin production. If the anaemia was severe, particularly if the boy has breathlessness, I would cautiously give a blood transfusion — this must be done slowly, in order to avoid fluid overload. In the long-term, erythropoietin can be given regularly to keep the haemoglobin above 11 g/dl, so avoiding the risks of repeated transfusions.

Other endocrine problems that occur in chronic renal failure are *renal osteodystrophy* and growth failure. Vitamin D is metabolised to its active form in the kidney, so there is reduced calcium absorption in renal failure, which leads to low plasma calcium and high plasma phosphate levels. This can cause pain and bone deformity. Treatment with vitamin D should be given to those children with a reduced glomerular filtration rate. It may be necessary to start calcium supplements and dietary phosphate restriction in established bone disease.

Growth failure in chronic renal failure is due to poor nutrition, uraemia, metabolic acidosis, and bone disease. Growth hormone is licensed for use in the treatment of children with chronic renal failure.

Q. When would you consider dialysis?

Dialysis is useful in acute renal failure; in patients with irreversible renal insufficiency; or when renal function is deteriorating. Renal replacement therapy may be by *continuous ambulatory peritoneal dialysis*, which has the advantage of being managed predominantly in the home, or by *haemodialysis*. Children with end-stage renal failure should be considered for *renal transplantation*.

HAEMATURIA

Q. What are the causes of haematuria in children?

Dipstick-positive haematuria is common in paediatrics. The sticks are very sensitive and in all cases I would want formal microscopy of the urine, both to confirm the presence of RBCs and to look at red cell morphology. Haematuria from the upper renal tract will show dysmorphic red cells; bleeding from the lower renal tract will show normal red cells. It is important to remember that some food stuffs, e.g. beetroot, and certain drugs, e.g. rifampicin, may colour the urine.

The major *causes* of haematuria are:

1. *Urinary tract infection*
2. *Nephritis*
   — Henoch-Schönlein purpura
   — post-infectious glomerulonephritis
   — IgA nephropathy
   — Alport's syndrome
   — nephrotic syndrome
3. *Renal stone*
4. *Trauma*
5. *Haematological*
   — coagulopathies: HUS, ITP
   — sickle cell disease
6. *Anatomical* causes
   — polycystic/multicystic kidneys
   — tumours
7. *Drugs*
   — cyclophosphamide
   — aspirin
8. *Recurrent benign haematuria* (diagnosis of exclusion)
9. *Normal*
   — post-exercise
   — menstrual contamination

Q. How would you investigate a child with haematuria?

I would want to take a history, examine the child, and do some baseline investigations.

From the *history* I would particularly want to know about the following:

1. Urinary tract infection symptoms — dysuria, frequency, urgency
2. Previous history of haematuria
3. History of trauma
4. History of preceding illness — URTI, diarrhoea
5. Family history of deafness — Alport's syndrome (autosomal dominant)

I would make a full *examination* of the child with special attention to-

1. Blood pressure
2. The presence of peripheral oedema, or ascites
3. Abdominal mass
4. Rashes — vasculitis, HSP

Investigations I would perform include:

1. Urine microscopy and culture — in all cases
2. Biochemistry — urea and creatinine, albumin, calcium
3. Haematology — FBC, film and coagulation screen
4. Renal ultrasound scan
5. Other investigations if nephritis suspected — ANF, ASOT, complement, hepatitis-B surface antigen
6. Other investigations:
   — renal biopsy
   — radionucleotide scans
   — urine calcium/creatinine ratio
   — cystoscopy
   — intravenous pyelogram

Treatment and prognosis depend on the cause.

HAEMOLYTIC URAEMIC SYNDROME

Q. What is haemolytic uraemic syndrome?

Haemolytic uraemic syndrome (HUS) comprises the triad of microangiopathic haemolytic anaemia, thrombocytopenia, and renal failure. It is the most common cause of acute renal failure in the USA and Western Europe. It is a systemic disease and, as well as the kidneys, it may affect the neurological system, with seizures and altered conscious level, and the gastrointestinal system. Two different clinical types are recognised:

1. *D+HUS (diarrhoea-positive)*: Associated with prodromal diarrhoea and is the most common type seen. It tends to affect infants and young children during the summer months. Many infectious agents have been implicated, including coxsackie virus, *Shigella* and *S. pneumoniae* but the majority of patients have evidence of exposure to verotoxin (a *Shigella*-like toxin)-producing *Escherichia coli* (VTEC). The most common serotype isolated is 0157:H7. Children present with pallor, oliguria and bloody diarrhoea. Hypertension and neurological involvement are rare.
2. *D–HUS (diarrhoea-negative)*: This form is less common, tends to affect older children and occurs at any time of the year. Predisposing factors include the oral contraceptive pill, chemotherapy, and organ and bone marrow failure. Neurological involvement is common.

Q. What do you know about the pathogenesis of haemolytic uraemic syndrome?

Vascular endothelial damage is central to the pathogenesis of HUS. The pivotal step in the initiation of cell injury is thought to be the binding of toxin to the Gb_3 (globotriaosylceramide) receptor of the endothelium, resulting in endocytosis and disruption of RNA transcription and cell death. D+ HUS is a systemic disease associated with activation of many inflammatory cytokines, including TNF-α, IL- 1α, IL-1β and IL-8. It is the thrombotic occlusion of small blood vessels that causes the microangiopathic disorder.

Q. How would you investigate a child with suspected HUS?

I would perform a full blood count, which I would expect to show microangiopathic haemolytic anaemia with fragmented red blood cells, raised WCC and thrombocytopenia. Platelet dysfunction is seen, with impaired platelet aggregation in response to agonists. Routine biochemistry reveals evidence of renal impairment with raised urea, creatinine, potassium and phosphate. Urine dipstick would reveal proteinuria and microscopic haematuria. I would send stool for culture for *E.coli* 0157:H7, although there are now more rapid enzyme immunoassays available.

Q. How would you treat a child with HUS?

Children with HUS should be managed in a paediatric nephrology unit. It is essential to maintain *strict fluid balance*, with fluid restriction and daily weights. Children with rising urea or potassium, oliguria, or fluid overload should be started on dialysis. *Peritoneal dialysis* is the method of choice. *Anaemia* should be carefully corrected. There is no evidence that anticoagulation or antifibrinolytic agents are of any benefit. The role of antibiotics in the prevention or amelioration of HUS is as yet unproven. Clinical trials are underway of SYNSORB Pk, an orally administered synthetic molecule that binds Shiga toxin within the lumen of the gut.

Q. What is the prognosis in HUS?

D+ HUS patients have a better outcome than those with D–HUS. Other factors associated with a poor prognosis include WCC $>20 \times 10^9$/L, older age at onset, anuria for >14 days, and severe neurological involvement. The acute fatality rate is 4–12%. Forty percent of patients continue to have some evidence of renal impairment and for this reason children should continue to be reviewed with urine testing, and renal function and blood pressure monitoring for life.

REFERENCE
Trachtman H, Christen E 1999 Pathogenesis, treatment, and therapeutic trials in hemolytic uremic syndrome. Curr Opin Pediatr 11: 162–168

NEPHROTIC SYNDROME

Q. What is the nephrotic syndrome?

The defining features of nephrotic syndrome are:

1. Proteinuria — urine protein $> 40\,mg/h/m^2$
   — urinary protein : creatinine ratio $> 200\,mg/mmol$
2. Hypoalbuminaemia — serum albumin $< 25\,mg/L$
3. Oedema
4. Hyperlipidaemia

Proteinuria results from a loss of negative charge on the glomerular basement membrane. Albumin leaks from the circulation, resulting in a reduction in the plasma oncotic pressure and loss of fluid from the circulation into the interstitial space, causing oedema. Hyperlipidaemia occurs as a result of excessive production by the liver associated with decreased lipid catabolism due to decreased levels of lipoprotein lipase.

In childhood the majority of cases show three histological changes:

1. Minimal change glomerulonephritis — 85%
2. Focal segmental glomerulonephritis — 10%
3. Mesangiocapillary glomerulonephritis — 5%

Classification is more usually divided into whether or not the condition responds to steroids as the majority of children do not have a renal biopsy performed.

Q. Tell me about steroid-responsive and steroid-resistant types of nephrotic syndrome.

Steroid-responsive nephrotic syndrome is of unknown aetiology and 85% of patients have minimal-change glomerulonephritis with retraction of the epithelial-cell foot processes seen on electron microscopy. It has an incidence of 1:5000 and usually occurs in 2-6-year-olds, with a male to female ratio of 2:1. It is often preceded by an upper respiratory tract infection. Ninety percent of these children respond to oral prednisolone within 28 days. Seventy-five percent will relapse at least once after stopping or reducing the steroid. Some children become dependent on steroids to maintain remission.

Children with *steroid-resistant nephrotic syndrome* do not respond to oral steroids within 28 days. This can often be predicted from the outset by the age of onset (<6 months or >12 years); the presence of gross haematuria; and persistent microscopic haematuria associated with hypertension and/or low plasma C3. These children should undergo a renal biopsy at diagnosis and be under the care of a paediatric nephrologist.

Q. How would you investigate a child with suspected nephrotic syndrome?

Investigations can be divided into blood tests, urine tests, and renal biopsy.

a) *Blood tests*:
   — FBC
   — urea and electrolytes
   — albumin
   — hepatitis B antigen
   — varicella antibody titre
   — lipids/cholesterol
   — ASOT
   — complement
   — ANF
b) *Urine tests*:
   — urine microscopy and culture
   — early morning protein : creatinine ratio (>200 mg/mmol)
c) *Renal biopsy*:
   — for steroid-resistant disease
   — atypical clinical features

Q. What are the major complications of nephrotic syndrome?

The complications of nephrotic syndrome include:

1. *Infection*. Nephrotic children are prone to infection, due to low IgG levels, impaired lymphocyte function, and the effect of steroids. They are particularly susceptible to *Streptococcus pneumoniae* peritonitis and for that reason children should be given prophylactic penicillin. The normal vaccinations should be given and the current recommendation is that they receive pneumococcal and *Haemophilus influenzae* vaccinations. Vaccinations should not be given until the child has been off immunosuppression for 3 months and live vaccines are contraindicated unless the child has had only a low dose of oral prednisolone (< 0.5 mg/kg/alternate day) in the previous 3 months.

   Varicella-non-immune children who have received immunosuppressive therapy within the previous 3 months should be given varicella immunoglobulin if they are in contact with chickenpox and should be given aciclovir if they develop chickenpox.

2. *Thrombosis*. These children are hypercoagulable, due to elevated clotting factors and enhanced platelet aggregation. *Renal vein thrombosis* is a particular problem.

3. *Hypovolaemia*. Often seen at presentation and during relapses. Children with significant hypovolaemia should be resuscitated with 10–20 ml/kg of 4.5% HAS. Those with severe oedema or ascites can be given 1g/kg (5 ml/kg) of 20% HAS, followed by 1 mg/kg of furosemide (frusemide) to promote fluid loss from the 3rd space.

4. *Side-effects of treatment*. side-effects of prolonged steroid use are common.

Q. How would you manage a child newly diagnosed with nephrotic syndrome?

Once the child was adequately resuscitated and the investigations performed as outlined earlier, I would manage the child as follows:

a) *Diet*. A well-balanced diet with no added salt.
b) *Fluids*. Avoidance of excess fluid intake. If severe oedema is present, restrict fluids to 1000 ml/m^2/24 hours. If fluid retention is severe, diuretics furosemide (frusemide) and spironolactone should be considered.
c) *Steroids*:

i)	Initial episode.	Prednisolone 60 mg/kg/m^2/day (max 80 mg/day) until remission (i.e. no proteinuria), followed by 40 mg/kg/m^2 (max 60 mg/day) on alternate days for 4 weeks.
ii)	First two relapses.	Prednisolone 60 mg/kg/m^2/day (max 80 mg/day) until remission, followed by 40 mg/kg/m^2 (max 60 mg/day) on alternate days for 4 weeks.
iii)	Frequent relapses.	Maintenance prednisolone 0.1–0.5 mg/kg alternate days for 3–6 months, then reduce.

   iv) Relapse on prednisolone >0.5 mg/kg/alternate days. Levamisole 2.5 mg/kg alternate days for 4–12 months.
   v) Relapse on prednisolone >0.5 mg/kg/alternate days and steroid side-effects or risk factors, or relapse on prednisolone >1 mg/kg/alternate days. Cyclophosphamide 3 mg/kg/day for 8 weeks.
   vi) Post-cyclophosphamide relapses. As ii) and iii) above.
   vii) Relapse on prednisolone >0.5 mg/kg/alternate days. Cyclosporin 5 mg/kg/day for 1 year.

It is essential that parents are taught how to dipstick urine.
NB. Relapse = 3+ proteinuria for 3 days or 2+ proteinuria for 10 days.

Q. What is the prognosis in nephrotic syndrome?

There are no predictors of this, but at least 60–75% will relapse. Parents should test the urine every morning for proteinuria and if there is 3+ proteinuria for 3 days or 2+ proteinuria for 10 days they should seek medical advice.

Children on long-term steroids should be assessed regularly for growth and blood-pressure measurement, and checked annually for the development of subcapsular cataracts.

REFERENCES
Evans J H C 1997 Current management of nephrotic syndrome. Curr Paediatr 7: 32–35
Hogg R J et al 2000 Evaluation and management of proteinuria and nephrotic syndrome in children. Pediatrics 105: 1242–1249

Q. How would you manage a child newly diagnosed with

Neurology

7

CREUTZFELDT-JAKOB DISEASE

Q. What can you tell us about Creutzfeldt-Jakob disease?

Creutzfeldt-Jakob disease (CJD) was first described in the 1920s and is a form of transmissible spongiform encephalopathy (TSE). TSEs are believed to be caused by proteinaceous infectious particles (*prions*). CJD classically affects older adults (> 60 years of age) with an equal sex incidence. It presents with rapidly progressing dementia, myoclonus, pyramidal and extrapyramidal dysfunction, spasticity, and behavioural changes. The EEG is typically abnormal. It is usually fatal within 12 months of onset of symptoms. In the majority of CJD cases there is no known cause but it does occur in sporadic, iatrogenic and familial forms.

The *sporadic* form accounts for 85% of cases. The exact cause is unknown but an age-related mutation of the prion protein gene has been proposed. No association with blood transfusion or consumption of meat has been identified.

The *familial* form accounts for around 10% of cases. An association with a mutation at codon 200 of the prion protein gene has been found.

Iatrogenic forms are rare but associated with the use of contaminated human growth hormone, contaminated EEG electrodes, neurosurgical electrodes, dura mater grafts, and infected corneal grafts.

Q. What is new variant Creutzfeldt-Jakob disease?

New variant Creutzfeldt-Jakob disease (nv-CJD) was first described in 1996. It is distinguishable from classical CJD in that it typically affects younger adults (aged 16–40 years), with classical neuropathology (PrP plaque surrounded by a halo of spongiform change) and a non-diagnostic or normal EEG. The clinical presentation is different from classical CJD in that the initial symptoms tend to be psychiatric, followed by the development of ataxia and myoclonus. Death usually occurs after 12 months. Nv-CJD and bovine

PASS ✓

spongiform encephalopathy (BSE) in cattle are believed to be caused by the same prion and nv-CJD is believed to be the human manifestation of BSE.

Q. Tell us about nv-CJD and blood transfusion.

It is still unclear whether nv-CJD can be spread by blood products. If it is, leucocytes would be the most likely source of infectivity. Given this uncertainty, in 1998 the Department of Health stated that all blood in the UK should be subjected to leucodepletion and that plasma products should be manufactured from non-UK-sourced plasma. The concern over blood products was increased further in 1999 when the US Food and Drug Administration (FDA) imposed a ban on blood donations from anyone who had spent more than 6 months in Britain during the years from 1980 to 1997.

REFERENCES
Collinge J 1999 Variant Creutzfeldt-Jakob disease. Lancet 354: 317–323
Turner M L 1999 The impact of new-variant Creutzfeldt-Jakob disease on blood
    transfusion practice. Br J Haematol 106: 842–850

CEREBRAL PALSY

Q. What is your definition of cerebral palsy?

Cerebral palsy is a disorder of movement and posture due to non-progressive brain damage sustained by the immature brain. It is persistent but not static and the clinical features evolve throughout childhood. Although the term 'cerebral palsy' describes purely motor dysfunction, other parts of the brain may be affected by the same pathological process, and associated features include epilepsy, cognitive impairment, and visual and hearing impairment.

Q. Who do you think should be involved in the management of a child with cerebral palsy?

Cerebral palsy is a complex disorder and should be managed by a multidisciplinary team. Throughout childhood regular assessments are essential as the pattern of motor deficit and the needs of the child change with time. Important members of the team include the physiotherapist, occupational therapist, social worker, speech therapist, dietician, audiologist, ophthalmologist, orthopaedic surgeon, and paediatrician.

The *physiotherapist* will work closely with the child and the family. The effectiveness of early physiotherapy in cerebral palsy has not been proven due to a lack of suitable control subjects. However, early physiotherapy and positioning are thought to be important for the prevention of contractures. The physiotherapist will have a lot of contact with the child and an important role in teaching the family how to handle the child in all aspects of daily living. The physiotherapist will teach the family exercises that can be done at home.

The *occupational therapist* in the team will assess the child with respect to the activities of everyday living. Changes to the family home may be required to enable the child to be more independent, for example ramps for wheelchairs, and special cutlery. Some children with cerebral palsy may have sensory deficits and the occupational therapist may be able to devise a sensory stimulation programme to accelerate the child's learning.

The *social worker* will be able to suggest benefits that the family may be entitled to claim. They can be supportive in times of stress and may be able to arrange respite care for the family.

The *speech therapist* should be involved before speech develops. They can assess the child's ability to swallow and use the tongue and may be able to teach methods for inhibiting reflexes which may be preventing normal feeding.

Failure to thrive is a common problem due to inadequate nutrition. In many cases the *dietician* might recommend a high calorie diet and, if the child still fails to thrive, feeding may be achieved by nasogastric tube or gastrostomy.

Hearing and vision should be assessed by an *audiologist* and *ophthalmologist*. Squints are common and surgical correction may be needed.

An *orthopaedic surgeon* may be needed for the correction of contractures and to improve posture. Surgical intervention is rarely needed before the age of 5 years.

Planning the education of the child is important and the child should be assessed for a *statement of educational needs* once in nursery.

The *paediatrician* should coordinate all these professionals as well as attending to the medical needs of the child. These may include anticonvulsant medication for seizures, treatment of spasticity with baclofen, and laxatives for constipation. Regular review of the child will highlight difficulties as they arise.

Q. Are you aware of any new strategies in the treatment of spasticity in cerebral palsy?

There has been a great deal of interest recently in the use of botulinum toxin by intramuscular injection for the treatment of contractures in children with cerebral palsy. In 1995 a UK working party was established to investigate the role of botulinum toxin in these children. Children with evidence of hypertonicity, but without fixed contractures, were entered into the study. Neurological and biomechanical outcome measures included video gait-analysis and a clinical assessment of joint movement. The study was inconclusive. A recent Cochrane Review was also inconclusive. The results of large ongoing studies are awaited.

REFERENCES
Ade-Hall R A, Moore A P 2000 Botulinum toxin type A in the treatment of lower limb spasticity in cerebral palsy. Cochrane Database Syst Rev 2: CD001408
Carr L J et al 1998 Position paper on the use of botulinum toxin in cerebral palsy. Arch Dis Child 79: 271–273

EPILEPSY

Q. How do you classify epilepsy?

A number of classifications exist, based variously on clinical description, age of onset, EEG findings, anatomy, aetiology, prognosis and others! The International League Against Epilepsy (ILAE) uses a straightforward system based on whether seizures are partial, generalised or unclassified. Further breakdown into simple and complex seizures makes this a straight forward and commonly used classification:

1. *Partial seizures*:
   — simple partial (focal) epilepsy
   — complex partial epilepsy — loss of consciousness from the start of the fit
   — partial with secondary generalisation
2. *Generalised seizures*:
   — simple absence
   — complex absence
   — myoclonic fits
   — tonic-clonic fits
   — clonic fits
   — tonic fits
   — atonic fits
3. *Unclassified*

Q. How would you investigate a first fit?

This would depend on the nature and circumstances of the fit and, to a certain extent, the wishes of the parents and the child. Fifty out of every thousand children will have at least one fit during childhood. If it is a short-lived generalised tonic-clonic seizure and there are no worrying features in the history or on neurological examination, I would simply watch and wait. Thirty-five percent of patients will have a second seizure, over 10% within 6 months of the first. The risk of recurrence after two seizures is 80–90%. In routine practice there are three main investigative procedures — EEG, CT and MRI scanning.

EEG is a useful investigation but should not be considered a screening test, nor a 'blanket' investigation for all first fits. Ten percent of individuals with epilepsy will have a completely normal EEG and 1% of non-epileptics will have an epileptiform EEG. It is diagnostic for benign partial epilepsy with centrotemporal spikes (Rolandic epilepsy); absence seizures (3–4 per second spike-and-wave); and infantile spasms (hypsarrhythmia).

CT scanning is available in the vast majority of hospitals in the UK. It is useful in status epilepticus for the detection of generalised cerebral oedema and raised intracranial pressure, acute bleeds, tumours, and calcification.

However, it involves significant exposure to radiation and is not appropriate for investigation of a first fit in the majority of children.

MRI is considered to be the investigation of choice in children with fits who require neuroimaging. I would request MRI for any child in the following categories:

— afebrile seizures and status in the first year of life
— all children with focal neurological signs
— all children with partial (focal) seizures, except BPEC
— intractable and worsening seizures

Some might argue that it is every child's right to have an MRI scan after their first fit regardless of its nature. This is not practicable and a decision on whether to scan must be based on the likelihood of a positive result.

Other investigations are available but these remain largely research tools, e.g. PET, SPECT, and brain surface electrode EEG.

Q. What can you tell me about the genetics of epilepsy?

A genetic predisposition or aetiology may be present in up to 40% of patients with epilepsy. Greater levels of neuronal excitability may occur not only at different ages (i.e. febrile convulsions up to 6 years of age), but also in some families, as a result of a genetic tendency. Certain epileptic syndromes appear to display Mendelian or complex inheritance patterns. These include benign familial neonatal and infantile convulsions, autosomal dominant nocturnal frontal-lobe epilepsy, and juvenile myoclonic epilepsy. There are, of course, genetic diseases in which epilepsy occurs as a clinical feature, such as tuberous sclerosis, Angelman syndrome and neurofibromatosis.

By understanding the genetics of epilepsies we may gain insight into the pathophysiological cause of certain fits, for example the disruption of a specific ion channel. This may then guide us towards the discovery and development of more appropriate and specific treatments.

Q. OK, tell me about some of the newer anticonvulsants and their mode of action.

— *vigabatrin* — a GABA transaminase enzyme inhibitor
— *gabapentin* — a GABA analogue that is useful in refractory partial seizures
— *felbamate* — probably an NMDA receptor blocker. Blockade leads to an alteration in calcium permeability and voltage-dependent sodium channel function in the surface membrane of neurons. 1 in 2000 patients have a risk of either aplastic anaemia or hepatotoxicity and 1 in 5500 may die from taking the drug. It is used as an adjuvant in Lennox-Gastaut epilepsy and infantile spasms
— *lamotrigine* — ?blocks voltage-dependent sodium channels. It is used in Lennox-Gastaut and other refractory partial and generalised epilepsy syndromes

— *tiagabine* — a nipectic acid derivative that selectively inhibits GABA reuptake in the neurons and glia. It can be used for partial seizures, either as add-on or monotherapy

— *topiramate* — a sulfamate-substituted monosaccharide that blocks voltage-dependent sodium channels, potentiates GABA mediated effects, and antagonises glutamate. It can be used as an adjunct in partial seizures.

— *fosphenytoin* — recommended in the USA as second line (after benzodiazepines) in the treatment of status epilepticus. It has the advantage over phenytoin of being safe when given as a rapid i.v. bolus but is much more expensive

Key points

▲ Fits can be classified into partial and generalised, with further division into simple and complex.

▲ Investigation of a first afebrile fit would be considered appropriate for an infant if it was focal and if there are abnormal residual neurological signs.

▲ Every year there are new anticonvulsants being introduced onto the market. Basic knowledge of these is all that is required.

Tips

● No doubt the examiner has described a classification for epilepsy, hence the question – every man and his dog seems to have come up with a way of classifying it. The ILAE classification is simple, easy to remember and to non-neurologists is more than satisfactory. Our advice is to use it.

● Investigation of a first fit is a contentious subject. Try and use the politician's tactic of not answering the question directly, but describe the pros and cons of the various investigations available. That way you cannot be shot down in flames for an answer they did not want to hear!

REFERENCES
Pellock J M 1999 Managing pediatric epilepsy syndromes with new antiepileptic drugs. Pediatrics 104: 1106–1116
Robinson R, Gardiner M 2000 Genetics of childhood epilepsy. Arch Dis Child 82: 121–125
Wallace S J 1997 First tonic-clonic seizures in childhood. Lancet 349: 1009–1012

STROKE IN CHILDHOOD

Q. Tell me about stroke in childhood.

Stroke is rare in childhood, with an incidence of 3 per 100 000 and occurs most frequently in children aged 1–5 years. It is defined as a focal neurological deficit lasting more than 24 hours. If it lasts for less than 24 hours it is classed as a transient ischaemic attack. Approximately 50% of strokes in children are haemorrhagic and 50% occur in children with no previous medical history. The most common underlying systemic disorder predisposing to stroke is congenital cyanotic heart disease.

Q. What are the causes of stroke in childhood?

Stroke in childhood can be divided broadly into two major categories, ischaemic and haemorrhagic. *Haemorrhagic stroke* can be due to disorders of platelets, such as idiopathic thrombocytopenic purpura, or disorders of coagulation, such as haemophilia. *Ischaemic strokes* are more common and are usually due to embolic events.

Causes of stroke in children include:

1. *Trauma. Head injury* is the most common cause of hemiplegia in children, which may be due to subdural or extradural clot. A rapidly deteriorating child with hemiplegia may have tentorial tenting.

2. *Vascular malformations. Arteriovenous malformations* are the most common vascular lesions presenting with stroke in childhood. They are usually unilateral and 50% are in the parietal area. There is a high risk of haemorrhage. *Cavernous haemangiomas* are mostly supratentorial and in the territory of the middle cerebral artery. The capillary haemangiomas associated with Sturge-Weber syndrome usually present with epilepsy and rarely bleed. *Cerebral aneurysms* may be familial or associated with coarctation of the aorta, Ehlers-Danlos syndrome, or polycystic disease of the kidneys. *Moyamoya* is a rare condition of unknown aetiology characterised by narrowing of the large intracranial blood vessels and proliferation of the distal vessels. This results in the classical 'puff of smoke' angiogram pictures ('moyamoya' means 'puff of smoke' in Japanese). It is more common in children with coarctation of the aorta, Down's syndrome, and Williams' syndrome.

3. *Vascular occlusions.* The most common systemic disorder predisposing to stroke is *congenital cyanotic heart disease* although other cardiovascular disorders such as *valvular disease, cardiomyopathy* and *arrythmias* are also important causes of emboli. Other vaso-occlusive disorders causing stroke include vasculitis, dural sinus and cerebral venous thrombosis, sickle cell disease, and homocystinuria. Conditions predisposing to a hypercoaguable state, such as polycythaemia, severe dehydration, protein C deficiency, and protein S deficiency may also result in stroke.

4. *Infection.* Bacterial meningitis may cause hemiplegia through thrombosis of the cortical blood vessels. Post-infectious encephalitis due to mumps, measles and varicella may present acutely with hemiplegia. A cerebral abscess from a middle ear infection should also be considered.
5. *Ischaemia.* Status epilepticus, cardiac arrest, near drowning and acute hypotension may cause hemiplegia, but are usually associated with more global deficits. Temporary postictal hemiplegia may occur in epilepsy (Todd's paresis).

Q. How would you investigate a child with stroke?

Investigations can be divided into haematological tests and cranial imaging. *Haematological investigations* should include full blood count, coagulation screen, protein C, protein S, Factor V Leiden, and antithrombin III. It is important to exclude sickle cell disease by haemoglobin electrophoresis. The current *cranial imaging* techniques of choice are magnetic resonance imaging (MRI) and magnetic resonance angiography (MRA), although computed tomography (CT) is acceptable to exclude haemorrhagic stroke if MRI is not available. If the MRA is normal or equivocal in ischaemic stroke or if there is suspicion of moyamoya then conventional angiography should be performed. Children with 'clinical stroke' but normal imaging should have an EEG to exclude hemiplegic migraine.

Q. Outline your management plan for a child who presents with stroke.

All children with haemorrhagic stroke should be managed in a centre with neurosurgical facilities in case drainage or decompression are required. Acute seizures should be treated and the patient's temperature should be kept between 36.5°C and 37°C. Any haematological abnormality should be treated, following discussion with a haematologist, if necessary. Intravenous heparin should be given to children with prothrombotic disorders. Intravenous tissue plasminogen activator (tPA) should be considered for strokes that occur in hospital and are imaged within 3 hours. A multidisciplinary team, comprising physiotherapists, occupational therapists, and nursing staff, should manage all children with stroke.

REFERENCE
Kirkham F J 1999 Stroke in childhood. Arch Dis Child 81: 85–89

DEVELOPMENTAL DELAY

Q. A health visitor refers a 15-month-old boy with developmental delay. How would you proceed?

It is important to establish what sort of developmental delay is causing the concern. Broadly, there are four areas to consider when assessing childhood development: gross motor function; vision and fine motor skills; speech and language; and social skills. I would obtain a history from the parents to find out whether there is an *isolated* area of concern or whether there is a possibility of *global* developmental delay. I would also establish whether there had been any cause for concern during the pregnancy or at delivery. It may be necessary to retrieve the maternal hospital notes, as recall by the family may be confused.

With regard to *gross motor function*, as I take the history I would ensure that I ask about fairly early milestones first, so that the parents can feel encouraged by the progress made so far. I would expect a boy of 15 months to be mobile, either crawling, bottom shuffling, cruising around furniture or walking. If the child was not yet mobile, I would ask whether there was a family history of delayed motor development. I would be very concerned if he was not sitting unsupported.

If there was evidence of isolated gross motor delay, I would examine the boy for signs of abnormal tone, movement, or posture that might indicate cerebral palsy. I would also look for hypotonia associated with muscle hypertrophy, which might suggest muscular dystrophy. Other muscle conditions should be considered, such as myotonic dystrophy and glycogen storage disease, but these are much less common.

Fine-motor development is closely associated with *vision* and it would be important to make an accurate assessment of the child's vision, including examination for congenital cataracts and cortical defects, if there seems to be a problem with reaching accurately for toys. Similarly, *speech development* is dependent on *hearing* and a formal hearing test should be conducted on a child with impaired speech. I would expect a child of 15 months to have passed through the babbling stage and be making sounds mimicking adult speech. If the child has older siblings, however, he may be allowing the other children to speak for him, and be getting exactly what he wants by non-verbal communication — this is part of the normal spectrum of development.

In terms of *social development*, the child might be shy with strangers, but I would expect him to play contentedly with family and his peers. If this is not the case, it could be an early sign of autism, or of a more general global delay, as might be associated with degenerative conditions.

Q. So, what degenerative conditions do you know which cause global developmental delay?

Most of the degenerative conditions diagnosed at the age of 15 months are likely to be biochemical. However, if the symptoms or signs are of sudden onset, it is worth considering central nervous system infections, for example viral encephalitis.

The biochemical causes of developmental delay or regression are numerous, but rare. They include the *mucopolysaccharidoses*, such as Hurler's syndrome and Hunter's syndrome, in which psychomotor retardation may be associated with coarse facial features, corneal clouding, and skeletal abnormalities. Hurler's syndrome is inherited as an autosomal recessive condition, while inheritance in Hunter's syndrome is X-linked recessive. The diagnosis can be confirmed by finding the stored substances (dermatan sulphate and heparan sulphate) in the urine, and analysis of the specific enzyme defect after fibroblast or lymphocyte culture.

Lysosomal storage disorders also cause developmental delay, which may be associated with organomegaly or a seizure disorder. Metachromatic leucodystrophy is an example, in which sulphatides accumulate in the brain and kidneys. A CT head scan might show diffuse loss of white matter. It is inherited as an autosomal recessive disorder and can be diagnosed by identification of the enzyme defect after fibroblast or lymphocyte culture.

Tip

● Don't get carried away with rare diseases. Only mention those that you know a little bit about.

ATAXIA

Q. A 21-month-old boy has recently developed ataxia. How would you proceed?

I would start with an accurate history. An important feature to establish is whether the ataxia developed suddenly or had a gradual onset. The most common cause of *acute ataxia* would be *infective*. I would ask about fever and ear pain, as middle ear infection which persists can spread to form a cerebellar abscess. A recent history of chickenpox infection might suggest varicella encephalitis as a cause, but other viruses, such as Epstein-Barr and coxsackie, can also cause cerebellar infection.

Intoxication is another cause of acute ataxia. Alcohol ingestion is a possibility in a curious child of this age, but other poisons including drugs may cause true ataxia, for example phenytoin, or unsteadiness, for example benzodiazepines.

Very sudden onset of ataxia suggests a *vascular* event. These are rare in children, but a cerebellar haemorrhage from an arteriovenous malformation or a bleed into a tumour may cause ataxia. Basilar migraine can also cause ataxia and I would ask whether there was a family history of migraine.

One of the most important diagnoses to make is that of a cerebral tumour, either a *posterior fossa tumour* or any tumour causing raised intracranial pressure. The history might be longer in a child with a brain tumour and there is likely to be associated headache and vomiting if there is raised intracranial pressure. Another tumour which may cause signs of ataxia is a neuroblastoma, which is associated with jerking eye movements ('dancing eye syndrome'). However, this usually presents during infancy. Congenital abnormalities, such as aqueduct stenosis, may cause *hydrocephalus*, which occasionally presents at this age.

Progressive ataxia can be caused by many rare disorders and would be difficult to identify from the history. Few would present at this age, for example Friedrich's ataxia usually presents in early puberty and metachromatic leucodystrophy usually presents at school age. *Ataxia telangectasia* may present with truncal ataxia in a boy of this age. I would ask about recurrent infections, as children with ataxia telangectasia have IgA deficiency. The telangectasia may not become apparent in the sclerae until later in childhood.

My examination would include assessment of features suggestive of cerebellar pathology, such as nystagmus, hypotonia, dysarthria, and intention tremor. I would look for papilloedema as a sign of raised intracranial pressure and listen for a bruit suggestive of a vascular anomaly. I would also check that the boy had an ataxic gait, rather than an unsteady gait related to muscle weakness, as in Duchenne muscular dystrophy.

Q. So how would you investigate this boy, if we tell you that the ataxia has been gradually progressive?

I think that it would be a priority to arrange a head scan. The most urgent thing to exclude would be a brain tumour or hydrocephalus, as prompt treatment in the form of a ventricular shunt, or steroids when there is swelling around the tumour, might prevent further damage. A CT head scan would be adequate for this purpose, but an MRI scan would give better views of the posterior fossa. It would also show better differentiation of white and grey matter, which might be helpful in some of the degenerative causes, such as metachromatic leucodystrophy. MRI angiography might be used to delineate a vascular anomaly if this was thought likely.

If the head scan was normal, I would consider other investigations. An EEG is less helpful in progressive ataxia than in acute ataxia, when it might show encephalitis or non-convulsive status epilepticus. I would check immunoglobulin levels for evidence of ataxia telangectasia. I would also test for metabolic conditions, for example plasma and CSF lactate levels, which may be raised in mitochondrial disorders.

Q. Interesting. So tell us about mitochondrial disorders which cause ataxia.

The one I know most about is Kearns-Sayre syndrome. I recently met a patient with the condition who had ataxia associated with ophthalmoplegia and generalised weakness. It is caused by a defect in the respiratory chain, making energy production difficult at a cellular level. Some patients have high lactate levels.

Tips

● Keep it simple and remember that you can't include a fully comprehensive list of causes of ataxia — a list of diseases is not very interesting anyway!

● Don't mention mitochondrial encephalopathies unless you really know your stuff! Sound confident when you've finished, as the examiners will happily keep quiet and let you dig a deep hole.

Community paediatrics

8

NON-ACCIDENTAL INJURY

Q1. What injuries in a child would make you suspect non-accidental injury?

Non-accidental injury (NAI) is only one type of child abuse, albeit the most common. (The others include emotional deprivation, sexual abuse, neglect, and Munchausen syndrome by proxy.) It accounts for around 100 deaths a year in the UK and many more serious permanent injuries.

Abused children may present in a number of different ways and in a variety of settings — recognition is rarely straightforward. As always, clear and accurate documentation (and, if appropriate, colour photography) of the injuries is essential, including a detailed history of how the injuries were sustained, preferably from more than one person. Social and family circumstances and past medical history must be included. Relevant details of the *history* pointing towards a diagnosis of NAI include:

1. Delay in seeking medical help.
2. Inadequate, unrealistic or inconsistent explanation of the injuries, e.g. a 1-month-old sustaining a spiral tibial fracture by rolling over in her cot.
3. Inappropriate, indifferent or over-concerned attitude of the carer.
4. The accompanying adult being someone other than the parents, with no good reason why a parent is not present.
5. A history of previous injuries or attendance at casualty by the child or siblings, e.g. burns, scalds, ingestions, fractures.
6. An accompanying person unwilling to allow full examination of the child.
7. Child or sibling on the 'at-risk' register.

Features of the *examination* of importance include:

a) *Distribution and nature of soft-issue injuries.* The prevalence of bruising in infancy thought to be accidental in origin is about 12%. The more mobile the infant is, the more likely he is to have bruising over bony prominences. It would therefore be of concern to see bruising in a 2-month-old without reasonable explanation. It is extremely difficult for a child to bruise around the neck area as the head and shoulder protect this area very well. Bruising of different ages is of significance although aging bruises accurately is a very difficult area and is something that I cannot or would not do with any degree of certainty.

b) *Distribution and nature of fractures.* Fractures in under-ones are very rare and uncommon in under-threes. Greenstick fractures are much less sinister than spiral fractures of long bones. Metaphyseal chip or bucket handle fractures are highly suggestive of NAI.

c) *Highly suggestive injuries.* These include: bite marks; cigarette burns; torn frenulum; immersion scalds to hands, feet and buttocks; subconjunctival haemorrhages; fingertip bruises; and demarcated bruises and abrasions caused by belts, shoes, and the slapping hand of an adult.

Q2. OK, so you have a child who you suspect has NAI. How would you proceed?

As already mentioned, it is essential to get a detailed history from all parties and to have accurate documentation of all injuries sustained. The need for social-services input is essential early on — a 24-hour emergency duty team is available and if prosecution is anticipated the child protection unit needs to be involved. If there is a possibility of child sexual abuse, then joint (and single) examination is required with the police surgeon and I would seek the advice of my consultant on-call regarding procedure. Great emphasis is often placed on investigations with clotting studies and skeletal survey, but these are rarely contributory. The skeletal survey involves significant exposure to radiation and must not be undertaken lightly. If it *is* deemed necessary, it should be carried out during 'working hours' when specialised paediatric radiographers are available. Hospital is not a suitable place for a child with NAI unless medically unfit to be discharged and very often a child can be safely placed at home, providing the perpetrator is not present. Alternatively, social services may provide emergency foster carers.

My role would be to document the injuries and state whether the explanation given is satisfactory, rather than organise placement of the child. Almost certainly, a case conference will be convened in the near future and worthwhile input by the hospital paediatrician justifies attendance whenever possible.

Q. Tell me about some of the features of Munchausen syndrome by proxy.

I have been involved personally in a number of situations where the possibility of Munchausen syndrome by proxy has been raised and in a couple of cases where it has been proven. The perpetrators often show a number of the following traits:

— female
— a medical/nursing background (so able to provide a detailed history and fabrication of appropriate signs)
— attentive to the child's needs, virtually living in hospital with their child
— attempt to form close relationships with the staff on the wards
— a personal history of Munchausen syndrome themselves
— a lack of concern about the 'seriousness' of their child's condition

Proving Munchausen syndrome by proxy can be extremely difficult because of the deviousness of the perpetrator. Covert video surveillance has been suggested as a legitimate means of detecting it, although there are major ethical issues and considerable controversy surrounding its use.

Tips

● You would not be expected to examine a child with possible sexual abuse unless you had specifically been trained to do this.

● There is no shame in confessing to a lack of experience and seeking more senior advice in this area of paediatrics.

REFERENCES
Carpenter R F 1998 The prevalence and distribution of bruising in babies. Arch Dis Child 80: 363–366
Meadow R 1982 Munchausen syndrome by proxy. Arch Dis Child 57: 92–98
Stephenson T 1995 Bruising in children. Curr Pediatr 5: 225–229
Southall D P, Plunkett M C B, Banks M W et al 1997 Covert video recordings of life-threatening child abuse: lessons for child protection. Pediatrics 100: 735–760

ENURESIS

Q. Tell me what you know about enuresis.

Enuresis can be defined as the involuntary voiding of urine after the age of 6 years. The majority of children will be continent of urine well before this age, although up to one-third of 4-year-olds, 15% of 5–6-year-olds and 5–7% of 7-year-olds will have urinary incontinence. Boys have *nocturnal enuresis* more commonly than girls, whereas girls more often have *diurnal enuresis*. A child has *primary enuresis* if they have never been dry for longer than 6 months, and *secondary enuresis* if wetting occurs after a minimum of 6 months of dryness.

Q. What are the normal stages in the development of bladder control?

Babies usually void between 12 and 16 times a day. Bladder emptying occurs as a normal reflex when it fills to functional capacity because the infant has no ability to initiate or inhibit micturition. However, it is likely that the infant, and certainly the toddler, has cortical arousal with bladder fullness and voiding.

There are a number of processes which must develop before a child is able to gain control of voiding. These include:

— an increase in bladder capacity
— the perception of bladder fullness and impending detrusor muscle contraction
— the ability to initiate micturition
— the ability to inhibit reflex detrusor contraction to delay voiding, despite a full bladder
— control over the external urethral sphincter

There are a number of factors that impinge on these processes:

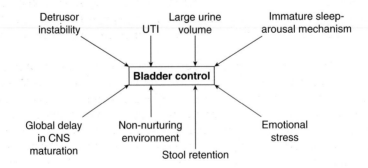

Q. How are you going to investigate a child with enuresis?

In all cases it is necessary to have a detailed history to define the problem; a thorough examination to exclude organic pathology; and a urinalysis to exclude urinary tract infection, glycosuria and a urinary concentration defect (random urine specific gravity >1018 = no defect). Further investigation depends on findings from the history and examination. For example, a 3-year-old who has never been dry and who has persistent dribbling of urine would require renal ultrasound scan, MCUG, and possibly cystoscopy to exclude a neuropathic bladder, whereas a child of 5 years with occasional wet nights requires no further investigation.

Q. OK, you think the child just has delayed maturation of bladder control — what are you going to do?

The most important factors in establishing continence of urine are the age of the child and the motivation of the family as a whole. Prior to the age of 5 years, I routinely: give patient and family counselling; correct any underlying

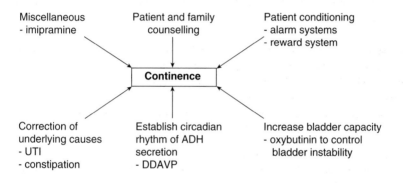

cause (e.g. UTI); restrict fluid intake within 3–4 hours of bedtime; and initiate a reward system, such as a star chart.

Alarm systems ('pad and bell', moisture alarms, buzzer alarms) can be used from around the age of 5 or 6 years. The proposed mechanism of action is the training of the brain to lighten its sleep stage or to relax the detrusor muscle as bladder filling occurs. Their principle drawback is that the majority of children with idiopathic nocturnal enuresis are deep sleepers and do not awaken with the noise of the alarm. Parents, however, usually hear the alarm and can wake the child to complete voiding in the toilet and assist in changing the sheets.

Some children with nocturnal enuresis lack the normal nocturnal surge in ADH secretion. DDAVP, a synthetic ADH analogue, can be used, either intranasally or more recently by tablet, to mimic this night-time rise and presumably decrease urine production during sleep. It appears to be more successful in those children with familial, rather than sporadic, nocturnal enuresis. Overall relapse rate (after initial success whilst on treatment) is high once the medication is stopped, but this treatment allows the child to gain continence for important events, such as scout camp.

The contribution of the various measures to achievement of continence of urine is difficult to assess because the vast majority of cases resolve spontaneously with time. I find that it is the children who have high motivation to

PASS
✓

succeed and who receive repeated support and encouragement in outpatient follow-up who experience the most successful outcomes.

REFERENCES
Chandra M 1998 Nocturnal enuresis in children. Curr Opin Pediatr 10: 167–173
Super M, Postlethwaite R J 1997 Genes, familial enuresis, and clinical management. Lancet 350: 159–160

CONSTIPATION

Q. Constipation is a very common problem in paediatric outpatients. How do you manage these children?

Firstly, it is important to understand what the family mean by the word 'constipation' — the child may be passing stools infrequently, or the stools may be hard and painful to pass. Some families consider an alternate-day bowel habit as abnormal. However, most children presenting to the hospital suffer discomfort when opening their bowels infrequently, which might be associated with abdominal pain or distension and often soiling.

95% of children presenting with the symptom of constipation will have no underlying cause. This is termed 'functional' constipation. However, it is important to rule out an organic cause, such as *Hirschsprung's disease*. This usually presents with constipation in infancy and may be associated with marked abdominal distension and vomiting. The disease is due to the absence of ganglion cells from the submucosal and myenteric plexuses in the large bowel wall and the degree of symptoms depends on the extent of the aganglionosis. The majority of children with Hirschsprung's disease will have been constipated during the first year of life and I always check whether the child passed meconium in the first 24 hours of life. The infant with Hirschsprung's may be failing to thrive and will often have an empty rectum on examination, while the child with functional constipation may have a reduced appetite, but will be growing normally and have a full rectum on examination.

Other *organic causes* of constipation include myelomeningocele, hypothyroidism, hypercalcaemia, and drug ingestion (for example, codeine-containing cough medications). These can generally be ruled out by the history and examination.

Most children presenting to outpatients with *functional constipation* have a longstanding problem. It may have started with painful defaecation, sometimes as a result of a fissure, which has led to a fear of bowel action, or in some cases with an acute problem such as dehydration. The chronic build-up of faeces in the large bowel means that the stools are in transit for a longer time and tend to be harder as more water is absorbed. Softer stool bypasses the hard stool and causes soiling. This can be particularly distressing for the child and needs to be dealt with promptly by *disimpaction*. Whenever possible, I prefer to do this via the oral route using sodium picosulfate. However, occasionally the child's degree of discomfort warrants disimpaction by enema and I tend to prescribe a phosphate enema. These should not be repeated frequently. Not only is it unpleasant for the child, but it can cause raised serum phosphate levels and dehydration.

The next step is to prevent the reaccumulation of stools. I start by giving practical advice, such as ensuring the child drinks plenty of fluids and eats a high fibre-diet. Diet is often a problem and it is sometimes difficult to find a high fibre-food product that the child will eat. I give a number of suggestions and find that a wheat biscuit cereal and fresh orange juice are the most popular suggestions. I also suggest that the child is encouraged to sit on the toilet for at least 10 minutes about half an hour after a meal. This makes the most of the gastrocolic reflex, which produces peristalsis when the stomach is full. It is important that the child is praised for this small step. Later he will need positive feedback for opening his bowels on the toilet.

In a child who has had longstanding constipation, it is difficult to prevent stool reaccumulation without medication. There are a wide variety of available laxatives, but I tend to use two. I use lactulose, which is a non-absorbable carbohydrate and acts as an osmotic laxative by softening the stool. I also use senna, which increases gastrointestinal activity — this is useful because the build-up of faeces causes the rectum to stretch, and tone will be improved by increased motility. I often use both laxatives initially, but tailor the dose to the child's needs by asking them to keep a diary. Although I start at moderate doses, the dose often needs to be increased. I always explain that because the problem has been long-term, it is likely to take a long time to resolve, and that the family should not worry about the child being on laxatives for a long time. I see the child frequently initially, mainly for encouragement but also in order to manipulate the dosage of laxatives. Once the child is opening his bowels easily I gradually reduce the medication over a number of months.

Tip

- Demonstrate your *own* experience whenever possible, thinking back to what you have done previously in this sort of situation. If you haven't already had the chance, make sure you go to some general paediatric outpatient clinics. This is the sort of problem you will see all the time.

ATTENTION DEFICIT HYPERACTIVITY DISORDER

Q. A general practitioner refers a patient whom he suspects may have attention deficit hyperactivity disorder. What would you do in your initial assessment?

In my experience, it is usually the parents who have noticed a behavioural disturbance in their child which they consider to be abnormal and the most important thing is to establish what features are worrying them.

The main features of attention deficit hyperactivity disorder (ADHD) are inattention, impulsive behaviour, and motor restlessness, but these features may be present to a variable extent. I would want to take a detailed history from both parents. Signs of *inattentiveness* might include being easily distracted and having difficulty completing a task. Features of *impulsive behaviour* might be a quick temper or suddenly getting up from the chair when doing work at school. The *hyperactivity* might present as fidgetiness or running about at inappropriate times. Many of these features are non-specific, but children with ADHD usually have features of the disorder prior to the age of 7 years. It is important to find out whether the features persist in more than one environment, for example both at school and at home. If the features are only present when the child is at home, this might suggest that the behaviour is related more to environmental factors than to ADHD.

During my discussion with the parents, I would try to involve the child as much as possible to see if he agrees with the description of his behaviour. I would also be watching the child's behaviour as this may give me more clues. However, I would not dismiss the diagnosis in a child who behaves immaculately during an interview, as he has only been observed for a snapshot of time.

I would examine the child for any physical disorder which might explain his symptoms, looking particularly for signs of deafness. I would then write to the child's school to ask for more information about his behaviour there, as this will offer further insight. There are questionnaires which have been developed for the assessment of ADHD and I have found the *Conners' rating scale* quite useful for a detailed assessment — this is completed by the parents, teacher and, where possible, the child.

If my assessment suggests that ADHD is likely, I would ask a colleague in child psychiatry to review the child.

Q. Assuming that the psychiatrist agrees with the diagnosis, how would you proceed?

The management of ADHD is difficult and I would be keen to share the care with the psychiatrist or a clinical psychologist. *Behavioural management programmes* may be effective to a certain extent, but these children do not tend to respond to boundaries in the same way as other children. The families will need a lot of support, which might come from their families, psychologists, or the national family support group. It is usual to try to identify some 'rules' which the child must adhere to and, meanwhile, to ignore behaviour which is not harmful to anyone. In this way the child is not being constantly rebuked, but understands that there are limits. It is also important to identify areas in which the child does well, for example sports or art, so that praise and rewards can be given appropriately.

Q. Are there any medications which might supplement behavioural management?

Centrally acting stimulants, such as methylphenidate, have been shown to be effective in placebo-controlled trials. They have a fast onset of action (within 30 minutes) and a short duration of action (about 3 hours). They therefore need to be given frequently throughout the day, for maximum effect when concentration is required at school. Some children use them only on school days. The dose needs to be increased gradually over a number of weeks. Unwanted side-effects include growth retardation and appetite suppression. As they are stimulants they may cause insomnia and are best avoided in the evenings. Not all children respond to a particular stimulant and it might be worth trying an alternative, for example dexamphetamine, if methylphenidate has little effect on concentration.

Tip

● Use phrases which suggest your familiarity with a condition whenever possible, such as, 'In my experience', 'I usually use'.

REFERENCE
Hill P 1998 Attention deficit hyperactivity disorder. Arch Dis Child 79: 381–385

CHRONIC FATIGUE SYNDROME

Q. How would you make the diagnosis of chronic fatigue syndrome (CFS)?

In 1991 the *Oxford Criteria* guidelines were produced to help in the diagnosis of chronic fatigue syndrome (CFS). These were reviewed in 1996 by a working party of the Royal Colleges of Physicians, Psychiatrists and General Practitioners, who considered the guidelines suitable for making the diagnosis in children and adolescents. The guidelines for diagnosis recognise fatigue as the principal symptom, which is of definite onset, is not lifelong, and must have been present for at least 3 months. The fatigue usually affects both physical and mental functioning. Other common symptoms include myalgia, arthralgia, and headache. It is essential when making the diagnosis to exclude chronic medical conditions that may cause fatigue, and psychiatric illness.

An important feature is the remarkable absence of constant or reproducible manifestations of physical abnormality, either on thorough general and neurological clinical examination, or on extensive investigation. Over the years, minor abnormalities found in complex investigations (e.g. muscle biopsies, enzyme studies and MRI scans) have been reported in adults. Parents or patients are often quick to latch on to these and may come to the clinic armed with original articles in order to lend 'organic validity' to these symptoms. However, the consensus medical view is that no consistent abnormality has been found on investigating these patients and that there is no convincing evidence for an organic causation.

Q. What do you know about the aetiological theories of chronic fatigue syndrome?

The aetiology of CFS is still poorly understood and is probably multifactorial. The hypothesis is that the 'normal' sensation of fatigue experienced during a transient organic illness, such as a viral illness, is maintained by a variety of possible mechanisms, which may be psychological (premorbid personality, low self-esteem, psychiatric illness) or social (family-, school- or peer-related problems). A common finding appears to be a perception of the child's underachievement, either by the child or by the parents. The role of depression is uncertain but is probably important.

The concept of 'abnormal illness behaviour' has been used to describe a variety of reactions, including chronic fatigue syndrome, which may present in the middle ground between medicine and psychiatry in which physical complaints do not appear to have an obvious organic basis. Parents often become so involved in their child's illness that they perpetuate it and will often express exasperation with the medical profession's apparent 'incompetence' in understanding or managing the condition.

Numerous infectious agents, especially viruses, have been implicated, including herpes viruses (especially Epstein-Barr virus), enteroviruses (especially coxsackie B), CMV, rubella, and hepatitis-A, -B, and -C viruses. However, despite extensive serological investigations, no causal relationship has ever been proved. Other unproven theories include immune dysfunction and cardiovascular orthostatic intolerance.

Q. How would you investigate a child with chronic fatigue syndrome?

The primary objective in the investigation of these children is to establish the diagnosis by excluding other possible diagnoses. Parents appreciate investigations being performed as this helps to reassure them that serious pathology is being excluded and that their child's symptoms are being taken seriously. However, it is important that the parents understand that normal laboratory investigations do not disprove the reality of their child's symptoms.

A thorough clinical examination is essential in all cases. It is important to exclude chronic organ dysfunction, immunological disorders, and chronic infections by performing laboratory investigations, including full blood count, U&E, LFT, CPK, TFT, inflammatory markers, immunoglobulins, T-cell subsets, ANF, complement, monospot, and viral titres. A small number of children with more severe symptoms may require further investigations, such as cranial imaging or colonoscopy.

Q. Outline briefly how you would manage a child with this syndrome.

I would recommend a multidisciplinary approach to the management, with input from the GP, child psychiatrist, paediatric physiotherapist, and paediatrician. The GP may have vital information about the family dynamics and may be better placed to engage the family in treatment. The psychiatrist will be able to instigate specific treatment if there is coexisting mental illness such as depression. The paediatrician should act as the coordinator for therapy. In many situations admission to hospital may be necessary to initiate therapy, especially if the child is housebound or has psychiatric involvement.

The majority of paediatricians would recommend a combination of graded exercise plans and cognitive behavioural therapies. *Graded exercise plans* involve defined and mutually agreed steps so that everyone concerned can work towards predetermined goals. It is essential that goals are realistic and are frequently reviewed. The child must keep a diary of rest as well as activity so that the level of exercise can be increased in a planned way. *Cognitive behavioural therapy* involves teaching the child strategies for overcoming the symptoms.

REFERENCES
Franklin A 1998 How I manage chronic fatigue syndrome. Arch Dis Child 79: 375–378
Rangel L et al 1999 Chronic fatigue syndrome: updates on paediatric and psychological management. Curr Paediatr 9: 188–193

IMMUNISATIONS

Q. What is the current immunisation schedule for pre- school children?

Up until the end of 1999, infants were given primary immunisation with diphtheria, pertussis, tetanus (DTP), polio and *Haemophilus influenzae* B (Hib) at two months, three months, and four months. The primary immunisations had previously been spread out over a longer time period, but the accelerated schedule ensures the earliest possible protection against pertussis and Hib at a young age, without compromising antibody levels. Since the end of 1999, vaccination against meningococcus group C has been added.

Immunisation against mumps, measles and rubella (MMR) is given at 12–15 months. The next immunisations come at pre-school age, when boosters of diphtheria, tetanus, and polio are given with a second dose of MMR.

Q. You mentioned the introduction of meningococcal vaccine. Tell us more about that.

The highest incidence of meningococcal infection is found in infants and young children. Infection may cause rapid onset of illness, with symptoms often non-specific until the classical rash develops. Mortality can be as high as 10% in childhood and young adulthood and research has therefore concentrated on finding an appropriate vaccine.

There are several serotypes of meningococcus, but the most common types to affect the UK population are groups B and C. At present there is no effective vaccine against group B meningococcus, which accounts for the majority of infections in the UK. However, vaccines against groups A and C have been developed. They are produced by the technique of conjugation, in which the polysaccharide antigen formed from the coat of the bacteria is attached to a carrier protein. Immunisation provokes a T-cell response, stimulating immunological memory.

Although there is a combined vaccine for groups A and C, infants are currently being given just meningococcal group C conjugate vaccine. Children under the age of 18 months do not respond to meningococcal immunisation as well as adults, so the antibody response and degree of protection is transient, lasting only 3–5 years.

Q. Are there any contraindications to immunisation with meningococcal vaccine?

Immunisation should be delayed in an unwell child with a fever. It would be contraindicated in any child who has had a severe hypersensitivity reaction to diphtheria or tetanus toxoids.

Q. Do you know of any other new vaccines which might be considered useful during childhood?

A vaccine against *varicella* was developed in the 1970s, but is not used currently in the UK, although it is licensed for use in the US. Varicella usually causes a trivial illness (chickenpox) but it can lead to severe complications, including encephalitis, pneumonia, and superadded bacterial infection, as well as causing severe illness in immunocompromised patients, including neonates. Herd immunity attained by the widespread uptake of varicella immunisation would reduce these worrying complications. It has also been shown to be cost-effective in Canada, where loss of earnings by parents taking time off work to look after their children with chickenpox has been reduced. I am not aware of any plans to introduce varicella vaccine to our current immunisation schedule.

REFERENCES
Department of Health 1996 Immunisation against infectious disease (incl. 0000 replacement chapter on meningococcus). The Stationery Office, London
Gershon A 1998 Varicella: to vaccinate or not to vaccinate? Arch Dis Child 79: 470–471

SCHOOL NON-ATTENDANCE

Q. What can you tell me about children who fail to attend school?

This is a complex problem and it is important for a paediatrician to realise that it is not an isolated issue but rather a symptom of a number of possible problems. I would divide these into four main categories:

1. *School refusal*. School refusal is responsible for 5% of paediatric psychiatry referrals. Non-attendance at school is a manifestation of an underlying neurotic illness or emotional disorder. There are three age peaks seen: 4–5 years (due to separation anxiety); 11–12 years (possibly due to a change of school or an irrational fear of school); and age 14–16 years (due to exams). These children are often loners, with a previously good school attendance record, who tend to stay in the home when not at school. They are often anxious on preparation for school and may manifest somatic symptoms (headaches, abdominal pain) as excuses for not going to school. They do not exhibit antisocial behaviour and have high academic standards. Their parents tend to belong to the higher social classes and are often overprotective and anxious themselves.
2. *Truancy*. May be defined as: school non-attendance as a manifestation of an underlying conduct disorder. It tends to affect older children, typically over 8 years old. Unlike school refusers, truants display antisocial behaviour and tend to stay away from home as well as school. Truants usually have a poor school attendance record and are non-academic. They tend to mix with other rebellious pupils and often become involved in criminal activity. Families may be unaware of the non-attendance at school or may be unconcerned if they are aware. There is an association with lower social classes and large family sizes.
3. *Genuine reasons*. These include bullying, perceived underachievement, difficulty with certain teachers or lessons (such as 'games'), or undiagnosed organic illness.
4. Occasionally, *parents* deliberately keep their children at home, for example to care for an unwell parent.

Assessment of school non-attendance requires thorough evaluation, including a careful history from the child, parents, teacher, and GP. Whilst interviewing the parents and child I would try to make an assessment of the family dynamics. I would want to know whether the child can be separated from the parents at other times than school mornings, and whether the child has any specific worries, or is being bullied, etc.

Q. How would you manage school non-attendance?

The management depends on the aetiology. I will deal first with *school refusal*. Children with school refusal have an excellent prognosis with the majority returning to school. The key to treatment is an early return to school. I would therefore counsel both the parents and the child and then set a definite date for return to school. It is important that the child is sent back to the same school if possible, for continuity. In some cases, a child psychologist may be required. In situations where I feel that the parents are closely bound-up in the problem, family therapy or cognitive behavioural therapy may be indicated.

Truancy is a far more difficult problem as it is closely linked with numerous other social problems and the prognosis is generally poor. It requires a 'comprehensive management package', enlisting all relevant professionals. In particular, social services may be required. However, many of these children continue to display conduct disorders and not infrequently end up committing more serious offences.

AUTISM AND ASPERGER'S SYNDROME

Q. Tell me about autism

Autism belongs to a group of neurodevelopmental conditions called the *pervasive developmental disorders*. The diagnosis is difficult, although specific diagnostic criteria now exist in DSM-IV (*Diagnosis and Statistical Manual of Mental Disorders*, 4th edn). It is characterised by: qualitative impairment in social interaction; impairment in communication; and restricted, repetitive, and stereotypical patterns of behaviour, interests, and activities. Onset is usually in the first year of life (although many are diagnosed later), the prevalence is approximately 91 per 10 000, and it is three times more common in males than in females. The aetiology is believed to be idiopathic although 10% of cases are associated with known medical conditions (such as Williams, Tourette's and fragile X syndromes). The increased incidence in males was previously thought to be due to linkage with the X chromosome, although this is unproven.

All children suspected of having autism should undergo a multidisciplinary assessment, including assessment by a child psychiatrist, a speech and language therapist, and a paediatrician trained in neurodevelopment.

Q. I will stop you there. How does Asperger's syndrome differ from autism?

Asperger's syndrome can be differentiated from autism because affected children have normal language development and intelligence. Social and behavioural abnormalities are seen, as in autism, but these are often at the milder end of the spectrum, explaining why these children are often diagnosed late. Males are affected more than females and are frequently described as 'clumsy'.

Q. What role does secretin play in the management of autism?

Anecdotal media reports have described dramatic improvement in autistic symptoms in children given secretin for the investigation of pancreatic dysfunction. As a result, thousands of children with autism were given this peptide hormone, although it is not licensed for this use and at that time had not been investigated in clinical trials. The absence of safety data did not deter desperate parents from obtaining the drug for their children, often from the black market. More recently, a large study of treatment with a single one-off dose of synthetic human secretin failed to show any benefit over placebo in the treatment of autism. Further studies of multiple-dose treatment are awaited.

REFERENCE
Prosser J G S et al 1997 Autism and the pervasive developmental disorders. Curr Paediatr 7: 158–162

EATING DISORDERS

Q. What can you tell us about anorexia nervosa in childhood?

Anorexia is an eating disorder that predominantly affects girls, but is increasingly recognised in boys. It most commonly affects girls around the time of puberty, but its incidence in pre-pubertal children is now increasing.

The cause is unknown, but there might be a genetic predisposition as there is a familial tendency, with studies showing an increased tendency to anorexia in twins. However, it is difficult to separate genetic inheritance from upbringing in these circumstances.

Anorexia is rare in societies remote from Western influence, suggesting that there is pressure in Western societies which leads to the condition. There has been a lot of concern about role models for young girls, both models and pop stars, who are portrayed as being successful and attractive because they are thin. However, there is no clear evidence that this causes eating disorders.

Girls who get anorexia are often high achievers, who seem to be striving for perfection. There is a greatly increased incidence in ballet dancers and gymnasts. Boys who develop anorexia have often been slightly overweight and sensitive to teasing about their weight.

Q. So, how would you recognise anorexia?

The onset of anorexia is often insidious. It tends to start as a failure to gain weight, but then leads to weight loss. The sufferer tends to avoid food and may exercise excessively. They may have a preoccupation with the calorie content of foods and express a fear of fatness. They have a distorted body image, seeing themselves as obese. Some girls will present with physical symptoms, such as abdominal pain or nausea, which they use as a reason for not eating. As they begin to lose weight they experience insomnia, constipation and cold extremities. On examination, the girl may have a low blood pressure, slow heart rate, and dry skin. They may also have pubertal delay, or amenorrhoea if puberty is more advanced. Blood tests may show dehydration, hypothyroidism, or hypokalaemia, particularly if laxatives are being abused.

Q. How would you manage the situation?

The anorexic may find that controlling their food intake is the only way they have of keeping control of their life. It is important to show the patient that, in fact, adults have now taken control of their health. One of the most difficult problems is that the patient will usually deny that they have a problem with eating.

The first step is to set a realistic target weight, which aims for a 'safe' weight. Feeding will need to be graded, so that the girl is not expected to eat enormous portions in the first instance. There has to be firm guidance from carers, and mealtimes may need close supervision. Excessive exercise should be stopped.

Occasionally, patients require admission to hospital if they are very dehydrated or experiencing hypotension. Whenever possible, this should be done in a specialised psychiatric unit where staff are used to managing this difficult condition. Family and individual psychotherapy might also be helpful.

Q. What are the features of bulimia?

Bulimia usually presents in girls *after* puberty. It is a condition in which the girl eats excessive amounts of high-calorie foods rapidly, and follows this with vomiting. The girl may seem physically healthy, with a normal weight. She may be experiencing depressive symptoms or feelings of isolation. On examination, there might be calluses on the back of the fingers from inducing vomiting, or dental erosions. Bulimia often follows an episodic course, with a high rate of relapse.

Clinical pharmacology and therapeutics

PRESCRIBING IN PAEDIATRICS

Q. When prescribing drugs for children do you always ensure that the drug is licensed for use in that child?

Inevitably, drugs are prescribed in paediatrics that are not specifically licensed for use in children (i.e. unlicensed) or they are prescribed outside the terms of their patient licence (i.e. 'off-label'). Many drugs that are in routine use in paediatrics do not have a product licence. A good example of this is parenteral nutrition, that has no product licence for children, although it is commonly used in paediatrics and neonatology.

In order for a drug to gain a *product licence*, the pharmaceutical company must submit an application to the Medicines Control Agency (MCA), based on clinical trials undertaken to investigate different dosage regimes, pharmacokinetics, and toxicity. A licence is granted if the MCA feels, on the weight of evidence, that the drug meets acceptable levels of quality, is safe, and is effective. Unfortunately, for a number of reasons, these clinical trials seldom involve children, infants, and neonates:

1. *Financial reasons.* The paediatric/neonatal market is small compared with the adult market.
2. *Practical reasons.*
   — great difficulties getting ethical approval, particularly for premature infants
   — the need for multicentre collaboration to gain sufficient numbers of patients
   — recruitment difficulties because of parents' reluctance to involve their children in clinical trials

Because children are not involved in the initial trials a product licence cannot be given for that age range. Any adverse event arising from administering unlicensed or off-label drugs then becomes the responsibility of the clinician rather than the manufacturer.

A number of articles in the literature have recently highlighted the problem of unlicensed and off-label prescribing in paediatrics. This is a particular problem in neonatal and paediatric intensive care units, where polypharmacy is an issue and the patients are inevitably more sick than the general paediatric inpatient.

The Royal College of Paediatrics and Child Health (RCPCH) has addressed this very sensitive issue with the publication of *Medicines for Children*. This lists the current prescribing and dispensing practices in the UK and lists unlicensed and off-label products prescribed in children and neonates.

Only licensed drugs should be used where possible, according to the manufacturer's recommendation, until pharmaceutical company clinical trials actively recruit infants and children in preliminary tests. Where this is not possible, and benefits outweigh potential harm, extreme caution and vigilance should be used. Any adverse events, whether possible or probable, should be reported immediately through the appropriate channels (the yellow cards at the back of the *British National Formulary*).

Key points

● Unlicensed prescribing and off-label prescribing (prescribing outside the terms of the licence, e.g. using higher dosage or frequency than recommended) is common in paediatrics.

● *Medicines for Children*, a publication from the RCPCH highlights the concerns about unlicensed prescribing in paediatrics.

● Until the pharmaceutical industry includes children and neonates in their preliminary trials of a new drug, unlicensed prescribing will continue to be a major issue in paediatrics.

Tip

● Do not own up to prescribing unlicensed or off-label drugs, although we all know that we all do it, either deliberately or in ignorance. Instead answer the question by generalising — the royal 'we' is far less incriminating than the first person singular in this particular instance!

REFERENCES

Conroy S, McIntyre J, Choonara I 1999 Unlicensed and off-label drug use in neonates. Arch Dis Child Fet Neonat Ed 80: F142–F145

Conroy S, Choonara I, Impicciatore P et al 2000 Survey of unlicensed and off-label drug use in paediatric wards in European countries. Br Med J 320: 79–82

Turner S, Longworth A, Nunn A J, Choonara I 1998 Unlicensed and off-label drug use in paediatric wards: prospective study. Br Med J 316: 343–345

Turner S, Nunn A J, Fielding K, Choonara I 1999 Adverse drug reactions to unlicensed and off-label drugs on paediatric wards: a prospective study. Acta Pediatr 88: 965–968

ANTIBIOTICS PROPHYLAXIS AND ANTIBIOTIC RESISTANCE

Q. When do you use antibiotics prophylactically in paediatric practice?

There are a number of situations in which antibiotics are useful as prophylaxis:

1. *Short-course prophylaxis.*
   — prior to MCUG
   —'kissing' contacts of children with meningococcal disease
   — prior to dental procedures or bowel surgery in children with anatomical cardiac defects
   — febrile neutropenia in the immunocompromised child
2. *Long-term prophylaxis.*
   — post-splenectomy (penicillin)
   — following acute rheumatic fever
   — under 2s with proven vesicoureteric reflux and hydronephrosis
   — recurrent UTIs (debatable)

There are also a number of *contentious indications* for prophylactic antibiotics:

   — flucloxacillin in children with cystic fibrosis
   — vancomycin for prophylaxis against sepsis in preterm neonates
   — the prevention of pneumonia in children with measles

A recent Cochrane Review suggested that antistaphylococcal antibiotic prophylaxis may be of benefit when commenced early in infancy and continued up to 2 years of age in children with cystic fibrosis. This may reduce hospital admissions in the first 2 years of life and reduce the frequency of additional oral antibiotic courses. I know that some cystic fibrosis centres adopt this policy, whereas others do not.

The use of prophylactic vancomycin in low doses reduces the incidence of nosocomial sepsis in the neonate. However, there is the potential risk of antibiotic resistance developing and so it is not current practice on neonatal units in the UK.

Measles causes more than a million deaths a year, most of these from pneumonia in children under 5 years of age. However, the evidence supporting the use of prophylactic, rather than selective, antibiotic usage in reducing morbidity and mortality is slim.

Q. You have mentioned antibiotic resistance. Tell me more about it.

Excessive and inappropriate use of antibiotics is believed to be one of the most important factors in increasing the prevalence of antibiotic resistance.

213

About half of all antibiotic use in the UK and the US is in animals, much of it for mass treatment or prophylaxis, and for growth promotion. This is of questionable benefit (for the animal or us!). A significant proportion of human consumption should also be considered to be of doubtful benefit. For example, using antibiotics for the common cold, otitis media and sore throats. For the vast majority, these illnesses are self-limiting, even if bacterial in origin or if secondary bacterial infection develops. A number of Cochrane Reviews have studied the appropriateness of antibiotics for these common illnesses:

a) For the *common cold*, in particular, the major conclusions were that those treated with antibiotics had a greater incidence of side-effects and that the drugs conferred no benefit over placebo.

b) For *sore throat*, antibiotics do confer relative benefits but absolute benefits are modest. These benefits include some protection against glomerulonephritis; a reduction in the incidence of rheumatic fever, acute otitis media (to approx. 25%), and sinusitis (to approx. 50%); and a shortening of symptom duration by about 8 hours overall.

c) For *otitis media*, antibiotic usage varies from 31% in the Netherlands to 98% in Australia and the US. They convey a small advantage in terms of absolute reduction in pain after 2 days (by 5%). Antibiotics may have an important role in reducing mastoiditis but this could not be confirmed by the review.

There are a number of specific *antibiotic-resistant organisms* that cause major concerns, particularly to the microbiologist:

— methicillin-resistant *Staphylococcus aureus* (MRSA)
— vancomycin-resistant enterococci (VRE)
— multi-drug-resistant pneumococci, *Mycobacterium tuberculosis*, *Salmonella typhi*

MRSA
Exposure to cephalosporins is associated with rapid acquisition of MRSA in the hospital setting. The prevalence of MRSA has risen in England and Wales from 1–2% in 1992 to 32% in 1997 (in reported blood and CSF *S. aureus* isolates). Reports of vancomycin-resistant MRSA in Japan mean that these organisms are now resistant to all available antibiotics. MRSA-colonised patients discharged to nursing homes rapidly cross-infect other residents.

N.B. 'VISA' is a relatively new term bandied about in the microbiological world and means 'vancomycin intermittent-level-resistant *S. aureus*'.

VRE
This is becoming an increasing problem in hospital practice in the UK where cephalosporins are readily prescribed. Enterococci resistant to all synergistic combinations of antibiotics are now being seen and a few isolates are resistant to all antibacterial drugs.

S. pneumoniae
There has been rapid spread, worldwide, of penicillin-resistant pneumococci in the last two decades. This has resulted in the use of third-generation

cephalosporins for empirical treatment of life-threatening disease, such as bacterial meningitis outside the neonatal period. Resistance to cefotaxime and ceftriaxone has, however, been reported and consequently some recommend the addition of vancomycin until the antibiotic susceptibility of the organism is known.

Q. How would you tackle the problem of antibiotic resistance?

There are a number of ways of dealing with this worrying situation:

a) The raising of professional and public awareness of appropriate antibiotic usage, through education.
b) Development and implementation of evidence-based policies for antimicrobial therapy in both community and hospital settings.
c) Limitation of over-the-counter availability of antibiotics.
d) Improvements in infection control measures to prevent nosocomial infection.
e) Measures to improve patient compliance, to ensure that prescribed courses of antibiotics are completed.
f) Reduction in excessive or inappropriate use of antibiotics in farming practice.
g) Development of new antimicrobial therapies, such as:
   — quinupristin/dalfopristin — a synergistic combination of streptogamins for clinically significant multi-resistant E. *faecalis* and MRSA
   — oxazolidinones — a new class of drug
   — new fluoroquinolones — grepoflaoxacin, trovafloxacin, moxafloxacin

Key points

▲ In paediatrics, prophylactic antibiotics are used: prior to invasive surgery, invasive investigations, or dental treatment in children with congenital or acquired heart disease; for immunocompromised patients (e.g. post-splenectomy.

▲ A course of antibiotics for the previously well child with a sore throat and/or common cold is not indicated. Their necessity in otitis media is debatable.

▲ Tackling antibiotic resistance must start at the grass-roots level, with doctors prescribing antibiotics only where there are clear indications of benefit over potential harm.

Tip

● This is another of those 'need to know', hot topics. Every day more multiresistant organisms are cultured from some human secretion or another and published in the medical literature as a cautionary tale. Doctors are notoriously bad at throwing antibiotics about like sweeties and causing the microbiologist to have palpitations!

Clinical pharmacology and therapeutics

An Aid to the MRCPCH Viva

REFERENCES

Arroll B, Kenealy T 2000 Antibiotics for the common cold (Cochrane Review). In: The Cochrane Library, Issue 1. Update Software, Oxford

Del Mar C B, Galsziou P P, Spinks A B 2000 Antibiotics for sore throat (Cochrane Review). In: The Cochrane Library, Issue 1. Update Software, Oxford

Galsziou P P, Hayem M, Del Mar C B 2000 Antibiotics for acute otitis media in children (Cochrane Review). In: The Cochrane Library, Issue 1. Update Software, Oxford

Shann F, D'Souza R M, D'Souza R 2000 Antibiotics for preventing pneumonia in children with measles (Cochrane Review). In: The Cochrane Library, Issue 1. Update Software, Oxford

Tackling antimicrobial resistance. 1999 Drugs and Therapeutics Bulletin. 37: 9–16

CISAPRIDE

Q. Should we use cisapride in paediatrics?

In 1998 the Committee on Safety of Medicines and the Medicines Control Agency stated that cisapride was contraindicated in babies born before 36 weeks gestation, for the first 3 months of life. Furthermore, they felt that there were insufficient data to support its use in children up to 12 years of age. The decision to ban its use in UK neonatal practice has been seen by some as over-cautious and without good foundation.

To answer the question of whether cisapride should be used in paediatrics, three important issues must be addressed:

— is it effective?
— is it safe?
— is it necessary?

1. *Is it effective?*

Cisapride is a prokinetic agent that stimulates oesophageal contractility, increases lower oesophageal sphincter tone, reduces gastro-oesophageal reflux, enhances gastric emptying time and reduces whole-gut transit time. It has potential benefit for conditions such as gastro-oesophageal reflux disease (GORD), constipation, encopresis, postoperative ileus, chronic intestinal pseudo-obstruction, and dyspepsia. There is a wealth of medical literature supporting its use, although there are a number of papers that suggest cis-apride is less effective in the preterm infant.

2. *Is it safe?*

There is good evidence that cisapride can increase cardiac repolarisation time (prolonging the QT_c interval) in susceptible individuals. Furthermore, a num-ber of drugs can enhance plasma concentrations of cisapride by interfering with its metabolism by the cytochrome P450 system in the liver. These include the macrolide antibiotics (erythromycin and clarithromycin, but not azithromycin) and some antifungal agents (ketoconazole, itraconazole, fluconazole and miconazole). There is also a theoretical risk of elevated plasma concentrations of cisapride in conditions associated with defective cytochrome P450 activity, such as immaturity (prematurity?) and hepatic disease. The important ques-tion, however, is whether slight prolongation of the QT_c interval predisposes an individual to arrhythmia, particularly torsades de pointes and sudden death. From its introduction onto the market up to the end of 1998, over 140 million courses of cisapride were prescribed in America and Europe. Only two cases of arrhythmia in America could possibly have been attributed to the use of cis-apride alone, when prescribed and taken correctly. Problems arise when it is prescribed above the recommended dose (0.8 mg/kg/day), when it is taken in overdose, or when it is taken with agents that enhance plasma concentrations.

3. *Is it necessary?*

For the vast majority of infants with gastro-oesophageal reflux the condition causes no problems and they 'grow out of it'. In essence, it is a parental problem (frequent clothes washing and the 'psychological trauma' of seeing their child vomit). For these, cisapride is usually not indicated. There are, however, infants with gastro-oesophageal disease who fail to thrive, suffer recurrent aspiration, or have a significant degree of pain from reflux oesophagitis. If other therapeutic measures fail (raising the head of the cot, thickening feeds, other reflux medication), cisapride may offer a useful non-surgical treatment.

Q. OK, what precautions would you use when prescribing cisapride?

I would:

— avoid the concurrent administration of contraindicated drugs
— not prescribe cisapride above the maximum dosage recommended
— measure serum potassium, magnesium, calcium, and liver and renal function, all of which can alter plasma cisapride concentrations
— perform an ECG prior to and 2 to 3 days after, initiating therapy

The first two measures are common sense; the latter two measures are more contentious and open to criticism of over-investigation. If prescribing cisapride for premature infants — when there are no other alternatives available — I would perform these investigations routinely.

Key points

▲ Prolongation of the QT_c interval is a recognised side-effect of the drug but its relevance in paediatric and neonatal practice is undetermined.

Tip

● Sitting on the fence has to be the best option with such a contentious issue as cisapride treatment for premature infants. You must realise that you cannot win! One examiner may criticise you for over-investigating, another for even *thinking* about prescribing it. If in doubt, try and steer the conversation to something less provocative, such as the choice of investigation for GORD or nurse practitioner prescribing in the future!

N.B. On 19 July 2000 the Committee on Safety of Medicines suspended the product licence for cisapride in the UK as of 28 July 2000. They reported, via the yellow-card system, that there had been 60 notifications in the previous 12 years of serious cardiovascular reactions (five of whom died) thought to be due to cisapride.

REFERENCES

Bernardini S, Semana D S, Huet F et al 1997 Effects of cisapride on QT_c interval in neonates. Arch Dis Child 77: F241–F243

Cohen R C, O'Loughlin E V, Davidson G P et al 1999 Cisapride in the control of symptoms in infants with gastroesophageal reflux: a randomized, double-blind placebo-controlled trial. J Pediatr 134: 287–292

Hill S L, Evangelista J-L K, Pizzi A M et al 1998 Proarrhythmia associated with cisapride in children. Pediatrics 101: 1053–1056

Markiewicz M, Vanden Plas Y 2000 Should cisapride have been "blacklisted"? Arch Dis Child Fet Neonat Ed 82: F3–F4

Shulman R J, Boyle J T, Colletti R B et al 1999 The use of cisapride in children. A medical position statement of the North American Society for Pediatric Gastroenterology and Nutrition. J Pediatr Gastroenterol Nutr 28: 529–533

VARICELLA IN PREGNANCY

Q. How would you manage varicella infection during pregnancy and in the neonate?

Varicella infection causes chickenpox, which usually follows a relatively mild course in young children. However, the risk of *disseminated varicella* is much greater in the neonate. The risk to a neonate depends on the timing of infection in the mother.

If the mother has been infected in the first 20 weeks of pregnancy, the fetus may develop *congenital varicella syndrome*, which has a high mortality rate and causes microcephaly and growth retardation in those infants who survive. Varicella zoster immunoglobulin (VZIG) should be given to women who are varicella zoster antibody-negative if they have been exposed to chickenpox during the first 20 weeks of pregnancy.

If an infant is born more than 7 days after the onset of chickenpox in the mother, he will not require VZIG because maternal antibodies will have been produced and crossed the placenta, protecting the infant. VZIG should be given, however, to neonates whose mothers develop chickenpox (but not zoster) in the period one week before to two weeks after delivery.

Infants who have contact with chickenpox during the first month of life are also at risk from severe infection if their mothers are varicella zoster antibody-negative. Infants in contact with chickenpox (or herpes zoster) during the first four weeks should be tested and, if found to be seronegative, they should be given VZIG.

Q. What degree of protection does VZIG offer?

The infant at risk may still contract varicella, but it is likely that the disease will be modified after VZIG, causing a less severe illness. However, there are still fatal cases following VZIG treatment, so it is important to warn the parents to ask for help if the baby is unwell or develops a rash — prompt treatment with intravenous acyclovir should then be started.

REFERENCE
Department of Health 1996 Immunisation against infectious disease. pp. 251–261.
The Stationery Office, London

DRUG INTERACTIONS

Q. What can you tell me about drug interactions?

A drug interaction is defined as an alteration in the effect of one drug by another, which may be deleterious or beneficial. Drug interactions are particularly important in the very young child; in severe illness or in organ failure (with renal, hepatic or cardiac impairment for example); or when introducing drugs with a narrow therapeutic index. Adverse drug interactions may be divided into *pharmacokinetic* and *pharmacodynamic*. Pharmacokinetics refers to the body's handling of drugs, i.e. absorption, distribution, metabolism and excretion. Pharmacodynamics refers to the biological effects of drugs, including their therapeutic effects.

Q. How are drugs metabolised?

The majority of drugs are metabolised in the liver. The most important enzymes involved in metabolism are the *mixed-function oxidases*, of which *cytochrome P450* is the most important. Cytochrome P450 is located on the smooth endoplasmic reticulum of the liver cell. Drugs are metabolised in two phases: *phase 1 metabolism* involves a change in the drug molecule by oxidation, reduction or demethylation; *phase 2 metabolism* involves conjugation of the products produced in phase 1 with glucuronide, sulphate, and glutathione, rendering them water-soluble prior to excretion in urine and bile.

Q. Tell me about pharmacokinetic interactions.

Pharmacokinetic interactions are probably very common in paediatrics but rarely of significant clinical significance. Drugs such as corticosteroids, warfarin and the oral contraceptive pill are metabolised by hepatic enzymes such as cytochrome P450 and when used in combination with *enzyme inducers* such as anticonvulsants (phenytoin, carbamazepine and phenobarbital) and rifampicin, their metabolism will be accelerated and cause therapeutic failure. In the case of the oral contraceptive pill this can have drastic consequences.

Erythromycin, metronidazole, chloramphenicol, isoniazid, and sodium valproate have *enzyme-inhibiting* properties, which may cause dangerous potentiation of other drugs, such as warfarin, phenytoin, carbamazepine and theophylline. With both enzyme inducers and inhibitors, the opposite pharmacological effect should be anticipated if the drug is withdrawn after a period of administration.

Plasma-protein binding displacement will produce a transient rise in the plasma level of a drug but this will be accompanied by a compensatory rise in metabolism or excretion. The steady-state levels before and after addition of the displacing drug will therefore be similar. This mechanism explains the potentiation of phenytoin by sodium valproate. Incidentally, this also accounts for the potentially dangerous displacement of bilirubin from plasma proteins in the neonate by drugs such as sulphonamides, which may lead to kernicterus.

Interference with renal excretion is clinically significant if the drug is water-soluble, so that a large fraction is excreted unchanged. There may be dangerous potentiation of aminoglycoside toxicity (VIIIth nerve damage and nephrotoxicity) with cephalosporins or loop diuretics.

Q. What do you know about pharmacodynamic interactions?

Pharmacodynamic mechanisms involve interactions between two drugs at sites of biological effect and may be usefully divided into synergistic and antagonistic.

Dangerous *synergistic* sedative effects can occur with any of the CNS-depressant drugs, such as benzodiazepines, tricyclic antidepressants, antihistamines, phenothiazines (and ethanol). Non-steroidal anti-inflammatory drugs reduce platelet adhesiveness and will therefore tend to potentiate the haemorrhagic tendency induced by warfarin. Potassium supplementation increases the tendency to hyperkalaemia induced by angiotensin-converting enzyme inhibitors. Diuretic-induced hypokalaemia will increase the risk of arrhythmias caused by digoxin.

There are several examples of pharmacodynamic *antagonism* such as vitamin K and warfarin, and β_2-agonists and β-blockers. A less obvious, but equally important, effect is the antagonism of bacteri*cidal* antibiotics, such as penicillins or aminoglycosides, by bacterio*static* antibiotics, such as tetracyclines.

Q. What do you understand by 'first-pass metabolism'?

First-pass metabolism describes the metabolic breakdown of a drug between the gut and the systemic circulation (via the portal vein), during its first pass through the liver. An orally-administered drug which has a high first-pass metabolism will have a low bioavailability. Examples of drugs which show high first-pass metabolism are β_2-agonists (salbutamol and terbutaline), analgesics (aspirin, codeine and morphine), prochlorperazine, clomethiazole, oral contraceptives, and mebendazole.

Q. What do you understand by 'first-order' and 'zero-order' kinetics?

The majority of drugs used in paediatrics are subject to *first order kinetics* of absorption, metabolism and elimination. In first-order kinetics, a *constant fraction* of the drug is metabolised per unit time and it can be predicted that a 75% increase in the dose of the drug will produce a 75% increase in the plasma level of the drug. Drugs with first-order kinetics have a constant plasma half-life.

Drugs with *zero-order kinetics* are metabolised at a *constant rate* independent of the plasma concentration of the drug. The rate-limiting process is usually an enzyme-dependent reaction — once the enzyme is saturated the level of the drug rises rapidly. The most important drug demonstrating zero-order kinetics is phenytoin.

DRUGS IN PREGNANCY

Q. Tell me about the potential adverse effects of drugs on the fetus.

The taking of medication in pregnancy is a particularly sensitive subject, which was highlighted by the worldwide reporting of thalidomide teratogenesis in the 1960s. Despite this, information on the risks of drugs in pregnancy is sparse and, for ethical reasons, has been collected in a haphazard fashion, mostly by the 'yellow-card' system. It is important that all paediatricians are aware of the potential effects of drugs on the unborn baby.

A commonly-used drug that does not cross the placenta (due to its large size) is heparin. All other drugs cross the placenta and have access to the fetus, which means that they have the potential to affect growth and development. The harm that medications may cause to the unborn child can be classified into teratogenic or fetal effects.

Q. Tell me about teratogenicity.

Teratogenicity refers to the potential of a drug to interfere with the process of *organogenesis* in the fetus. This occurs during the embryonic period and lasts from the 4th to the 10th week of gestation (which is the 2nd to the 8th week after conception). A number of drugs are known to be teratogenic from either animal study data or from reported human cases. Many more are not known to be safe and should be avoided in pregnancy until a sufficient pool of safety data has been accumulated from sporadic exposure. This applies to most new drugs.

Thalidomide was used as a hypnotic/sedative and is the best known of all human teratogens. Administration between 6 and 8 weeks gestation resulted in phocomelia (the absence of limb long bones).

Phenytoin is well known for causing the fetal hydantoin syndrome which comprises craniofacial abnormalities such as cleft lip and palate, hypertelorism, broad nasal bridge, hypoplasia of the distal phalanges and nails, growth impairment, and developmental delay. Phenytoin teratogenicity appears to be in part genetically mediated as it 'runs true' in subsequent generations and may affect only one of a set of dizygotic twins.

Sodium valproate induces neural tube defects in 1–2% of pregnancies.

Carbamazepine is generally considered to be the safest anticonvulsant in pregnancy and many epileptic women are switched to it if they are planning to become pregnant. However, rarely, it is associated with abnormalities similar to those seen with phenytoin. Epilepsy is a difficult problem in pregnancy and, generally speaking, the risk to the fetus of maternal fits is greater than the risk of teratogenic effects of anticonvulsants. There is also some evidence that epilepsy itself is associated with fetal abnormalities.

Warfarin is a small molecule and readily crosses the placenta. If administered in the first trimester of pregnancy it is associated with the so-called 'fetal warfarin syndrome', which consists of nasal hypoplasia and epiphyseal stippling, with hydrocephaly or microcephaly, and developmental delay. This occurs in about 15–20% of cases where there has been first-trimester exposure.

The *retinoids*, such as isotretinoin, are used for the treatment of acne. They are contraindicated in pregnancy because they can cause severe congenital abnormalities, including heart defects, cerebral and ocular defects, microtia, micrognathia, and thymic agenesis. Approximately one-third of early exposures will result in significant abnormalities.

The use of *lithium* in early pregnancy is associated with a variety of cardiac defects (8% have severe disease), including Ebstein's anomaly, which occurs in 3% of cases.

Diethylstilboestrol (*DES*), a synthetic oestrogen, can lead to vaginal clear cell adenocarcinoma in the female offspring of women who were given the drug in pregnancy in late embryogenesis.

Tetracycline causes yellow-brown discolouration of deciduous teeth and bones.

Methotrexate causes short stature and craniosynostosis if given in pregnancy.

Cyclophosphamide causes growth retardation and cleft lip.

Q. OK, I'll stop you there. Tell me about non-teratogenic damage.

Non-teratogenic effects or 'fetal effects' are related to damage to organs after they have been normally formed during the embryonic phase. Several drugs are associated with 'fetal effects' but may still be indicated if the benefits to the mother outweigh the potential risks to the fetus.

In the second or third trimester, *warfarin* may result in fetal intracerebral haemorrhage, microcephaly, and cataracts. Despite the potential adverse effects, warfarin is often used — outside the embryonic phase and the immediate preterm period (when heparin is preferred) — in pregnant women with significant thromboembolic risk. (Heparin is too large to cross the placenta but prolonged use is associated with a high incidence of maternal side-effects, notably osteoporosis and thrombocytopenia).

Sulphonamides in late gestation may compete with bilirubin for protein binding and cause neonatal hyperbilirubinaemia.

Prolonged use of *aminoglycosides* in pregnancy may lead to fetal ototoxicity in approximately 2% of cases.

β-blockers may predispose to intrauterine growth retardation, fetal bradycardia and hypoglycaemia.

Angiotensin-converting enzyme inhibitors are associated with renal defects and anuria.

Aspirin has been associated with haemorrhagic disorders and premature closure of the ductus if used in analgesic doses.

Opioid analgesics, if used in large doses around delivery, may cause neonatal respiratory depression, which will reverse with naloxone.

REFERENCES
British National Formulary 2000 Appendix 4 (Pregnancy)
British National Formulary   http://bnf.org/

DRUGS AND BREASTFEEDING

Q. What do you know about maternal drug therapy and breastfeeding?

The vast majority of drugs are excreted in breast milk but in amounts that are too small to harm the baby. Milk/plasma concentration ratios vary from 0.3 to 1.0 depending on drug solubility, pH, and dose interval. Most commonly-used drugs can be safely administered to a mother who is breastfeeding. In particular, penicillin, cephalosporins, most narcotic analgesics, insulin, methyldopa, commonly-used anticonvulsants (sodium valproate, phenytoin, carbamazepine), furosemide (frusemide), digoxin, and β_1-blockers are considered safe. Both heparin and warfarin appear to be safe but phenindione should be avoided because of the risk of neonatal haemorrhage.

Some drugs are, however, potentially harmful to the neonate and should be *avoided* or *breastfeeding discontinued* if administration is deemed necessary. Examples are:

— cytotoxics (cyclophosphamide, cyclosporin, methotrexate) — cytotoxic
— carbimazole — suppression of neonatal thyroid
— amiodarone — neonatal thyroid toxicity
— lithium — hypotonia and cyanosis
— barbiturates — drowsiness
— benzodiazepines — drowsiness and failure to thrive
— chloramphenicol — bone-marrow toxicity and 'grey syndrome'
— aspirin — Reye's syndrome and hypoprothrombinaemia
— laxatives — neonatal diarrhoea
— prednisolone — continuous therapy with >10 mg daily may affect the infant's adrenal gland

Tips

● Giving advice about maternal medication and drug ingestion and their potential effects on the breastfed infant is a common scenario.

● If in doubt, say that you would look in the appendices of the *British National Formulary*.

REFERENCES
British National Formulary 2000 Appendix 5 (Breastfeeding)
British National Formulary   http://bnf.org/

INHALED CORTICOSTEROIDS IN ASTHMA

Clinical pharmacology and therapeutics

Q. What are the side-effects of inhaled corticosteroids?

Inhaled corticosteroids have been used to treat children with asthma for over 25 years. They are of central importance in the management of chronic asthma, markedly reducing the frequency and severity of acute attacks. Their prophylactic effects significantly improve the terrible morbidity and mortality associated with this very common disease. The systemic side-effects of long-term oral steroids are well documented and many doctors have understandable concerns about the potential risks. In addition, many parents are deeply concerned about the mere mention of the word 'steroid' and many attend outpatients armed with printouts from the internet and probing questions.

In general terms, the side-effect profile of steroids is excellent in relation to their benefits and it is important that parents appreciate that the dangers to the child of *not* using steroids far outweigh the dangers of side-effects.

I would first like to consider *local side-effects*, largely to dismiss them as they are rarely seen in paediatric practice. Oral candidiasis, sore throat and dystonia are reported to occur in children but much less frequently than in adults. These do not seem to be related to the dose of steroid or the type of inhaler used. Instructing patients to wash their mouths out after using their inhalers is usually sufficient to deal with the problem. Younger children who use a mask should have their faces wiped after administration of the steroid.

It is the *systemic side effects* that provoke the most anxiety. I will deal with each of these in turn. The effect of steroids on *growth* has been the main area of concern. Unfortunately, studies have generally been complicated and inconclusive, for a number of reasons, including: the effects of asthma itself; the ages of children studied; the interaction of asthma, asthma treatment and pubertal growth; the type of study; and difficulties with compliance and practicalities of growth measurement. Using knemometry, it is possible to detect growth suppression in most children immediately after starting inhaled steroids. These effects are dose-related and have been seen with budesonide at doses of 200 µg, 400 µg and 800 µg per day, beclometasone at 200 µg and 400 µg per day, but have not been seen with fluticasone propionate 200 µg daily. The clinical importance of this initial suppression of growth remains unclear. Studies of the long-term effects of inhaled steroids on growth are very difficult to interpret although studies from the UK, America and Australia have reported that patients on long-term inhaled steroids have normal adult height as predicted by parental height.

If I was counselling concerned parents regarding the effects of inhaled steroids on growth, I would stress that, firstly, there is no doubt that poorly-controlled asthma has inhibitory effects on growth, at least in the short-term; secondly, the long-term data are generally reassuring; and thirdly, proper prophylactic control of their child's asthma with inhaled steroids should mean

fewer courses of *oral* steroids, which have definite risks. It is essential to monitor a child's growth in clinic and 'step down' treatment whenever possible.

Another concern about long-term inhaled corticosteroids is a theoretical predisposition to *osteoporosis* in adult life. It is widely accepted that systemic corticosteroids do reduce bone mineral density, predisposing to osteoporosis. Similar effects are seen in adults with prolonged inhaled corticosteroid use. However, there are no studies in children showing a reduction in bone density.

Another important concern is *adrenocortical suppression*. The hypothalamic-pituitary-adrenal axis can be assessed by testing physiological secretion of corticosteroids and the adrenal response to stimulation. There have been various reports of impairment, using these tests, with doses of beclometasone dipropionate of 400–1000 µg/day. However, clinical adrenal insufficiency has not been reported in adults or children secondary to inhaled steroids alone.

Posterior subcapsular cataracts are a specific and well-recognised complication of long-term oral corticosteroid therapy. However, a Canadian study found no association with inhaled steroid therapy in children, even at moderate to high doses. Also reassuring is the lack of evidence of significant disturbance of glucose or lipid metabolism in children on inhaled steroids. The easy bruising noted in adults on even low inhaled doses does not appear to be a problem in children.

It has been known for a long time that oral steroids can produce *psychiatric* and *behavioural disturbance*. However, with inhaled steroids, such side-effects appear to be rare in children and are confined to case reports in the literature.

Theoretical risks about inhaled steroids remain and it is prudent to ensure that the lowest effective doses of inhaled steroids are advised. Generally speaking, aerosol systems are appropriate for the more severe cases of asthma requiring steroid prophylaxis, and spacer devices improve local pulmonary delivery and also reduce both local and systemic side-effects. Mouth washing after inhalation may help to reduce the risk of oral candidiasis and may also reduce systemic absorption.

Children on inhaled steroids should have their symptoms, inhaler technique and growth reviewed regularly.

REFERENCES
Price J 2000 The role of inhaled corticosteroids in children with asthma. Arch Dis Child 82 (suppl ii): 10–14
Rao R et al 1999 Systemic effects of inhaled corticosteroids on growth and bone turnover in childhood asthma: a comparison of fluticasone with beclomethasone. Eur Respir J 13: 87–94

Oncology, haematology, and rheumatology

10

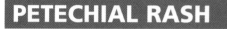

PETECHIAL RASH

Q. How would you manage an infant with a petechial rash noticed 6 hours after birth?

A petechial rash may be the result of a low platelet count or abnormal platelet function. My immediate reaction would be to assess whether the child was well or unwell. A well infant might have a petechial rash confined to the face as a result of the umbilical cord being tight around the neck at delivery.

However, the most common cause of a petechial rash at this age is infection. *Acute sepsis* might cause thrombocytopenia and disseminated intravascular coagulopathy, both of which can cause the petechial rash. If the infant had clinical signs of sepsis, I would immediately arrange close observation, do a septic screen and full blood count with film and clotting screen. I would then start antibiotics and consider fluid resuscitation. I would delay doing a lumbar puncture until the platelet count was known, in order to avoid the risk of causing haematoma around the spinal cord.

Congenital viral infections cause thrombocytopenia, often associated with hepatosplenomegaly and jaundice. I would ask about viral symptoms in the mother during earlier stages of pregnancy, then check maternal and infantile serum antibodies to rubella and cytomegalovirus.

Thrombocytopenia may also be a result of passive transfer of IgG platelet antibodies across the placenta in a *mother with idiopathic thrombocytopenic purpura* (ITP). I would check the mother's platelet count and ask about a history of ITP (even if the mother has had a splenectomy for ITP, the antibodies persist). *Maternal systemic lupus erythematosus* may also cause autoimmune thrombocytopenia.

Isoimmune thrombocytopenia occurs as a result of sensitisation of a mother who is platelet antigen-negative by antigen-positive fetal platelets. IgG anti-platelet antibody is transferred across the placenta and can cause thrombocytopenia lasting several weeks. Corticosteroids have been used when the platelet count is less than $40 \times 10^9/L$, but their value is unproven. The main concern is intracranial haemorrhage, usually occurring intrapartum

229

or antenatally in those infants at risk. Platelet transfusions can be given if the infant is actively bleeding, but the platelet count will drop again while antibodies are still present.

Leukaemia, usually the acute myeloid type, is a very rare cause of neonatal thrombocytopenia. It can be diagnosed by the presence of blast cells on a blood film and in bone marrow aspirate. The infant may have hepatosplenomegaly, and respiratory distress secondary to leukaemic infiltration of the lungs. Unfortunately, the condition is usually fatal in the newborn.

If the platelet count is normal, *platelet dysfunction* may be the cause of a petechial rash. However, conditions such as Glanzmann's disease, where the platelet membrane is abnormal, or Bernard-Soulier syndrome, where the platelets are large and have reduced adhesiveness, rarely cause symptoms in the neonate.

Q. So, now tell us what conditions you would consider if the same petechial rash was seen in a 6-year-old?

There are numerous causes of a petechial rash at this age. They can be divided into three categories:

— vascular causes
— platelet abnormalities
— coagulation abnormalities

It is usually possible to reduce the long list of possible causes to a more accurate differential diagnosis after a detailed history and examination. The most important diagnosis to exclude initially is *meningococcal septicaemia*, which usually presents with larger non-blanching areas of purpura, but can cause a fine petechial rash. If the child has been unwell with a fever, I would obtain blood cultures and venous access and then start fluid resuscitation and antibiotics immediately. In a less acutely unwell child I would ask about symptoms such as weight loss, lethargy, and mucosal bleeding, as I would want to consider *acute leukaemia*. I would also ask about *recent drug ingestion*, for example aspirin, which can reduce platelet adhesiveness. I would also enquire about a *family history of bleeding problems*, as milder haemophilias (e.g. Von Willebrand's disease) and platelet dysfunction (e.g. Bernard-Soulier syndrome) might present at this age. A recent history of diarrhoea might suggest the diagnosis of *haemolytic uraemic syndrome*, in which platelets are being rapidly consumed.

On examination, I would check the distribution of the rash. Petechial spots on the face might be the result of retching or prolonged coughing bouts in para-pertussis infections. *Henoch-Schönlein purpura* is usually associated with larger areas of intradermal bleeding, but could produce petechiae, classically over extensor surfaces, as a result of vasculitis. I would also examine for splenomegaly, which might occur in viral illnesses, such as cytomegalovirus, in leukaemia, and in portal hypertension, resulting in increased platelet consumption.

Idiopathic thrombocytopenic purpura may present with a petechial rash in a well child with a low platelet count. My immediate investigations in this child would include a full blood count and blood film, looking particularly for thrombocytopenia. I would also check a coagulation screen, which would show abnormalities in clotting factors. Other tests to consider would be bone marrow examination and bleeding time.

THE GENETICS OF CANCER

Q. Tell us about a child's predisposition to cancer.

Abnormalities or deficiencies in the genes that regulate cell growth, differentiation, or death may result in dysregulated cell growth and cancer. A child who has inherited, or acquired by genetic mutation, an alteration to their genetic make-up associated with cancer development has a 'cancer predisposition'. In 10–15% of all childhood cancers there is a strong familial association or the child has a congenital or genetic disorder that is recognised as having a higher likelihood of specific cancer types. There are a number of paediatric cancer syndromes in which these cancer susceptibility genes have been identified. These include hereditary retinoblastoma, Li-Fraumeni syndrome, familial adenomatous polyposis (FAP), multiple endocrine neoplasia (MEN) types 2a and 2b, neurofibromatosis types 1 and 2, Bloom's syndrome and ataxia telangectasia.

There are three types of genes associated with familial cancer syndromes:

— proto-oncogenes — cellular genes that, when activated, can promote cancer development
— tumour suppressor genes — genes whose loss of function causes cancer
— DNA repair genes — mutations may lead to inactivation of repair enzymes, causing cancer

Oncogenes
The most readily understood example of this gene type is the *RET* proto-oncogene located on chromosome 10, associated with MEN types 2a and 2b. Children with this mutation are at an increased risk of medullary carcinoma of the thyroid, phaeochromocytoma, parathyroid adenoma, mucosal neuroma, and gastrointestinal ganglioneuromata.

Tumour suppressor genes
Cancer predisposition resulting from inheritance of an abnormal tumour suppressor gene is associated with the development of tumours at a younger age than expected and in multiple sites within affected organs. This mechanism accounts for the majority of familial cancer syndromes, including familial retinoblastoma, neurofibromatosis types 1 and 2, familial adenomatous polyposis and Li-Fraumeni syndrome.

Retinoblastoma can be hereditary (40% of cases) or non-hereditary. In the inherited form the child has a germinal mutation in one copy of the retinoblastoma 1 (*RB1*) gene on chromosome 13. Malignant transformation of a cell occurs when the second of the genes acquires a somatic mutation. In the non- hereditary form the child acquires two somatic mutations of the *RB1* gene and tends to have unilateral (as opposed to bilateral in the inherited form) and later-onset disease.

DNA repair genes
Mismatch repair genes scan newly formed DNA, removing erroneously incorporated base pairs and reconstructing the corrected DNA. Functional

inactivation of both genes for the enzymes involved leads to tumour development. Examples of this type of defect are ataxia telangectasia, Bloom's syndrome and hereditary non-polyposis colon cancer.

Q. Which children should we test for cancer predisposition?

Before a child is screened for increased risk of cancer development, it should be considered whether this is being done in the best interests of that child. The determination of 'best interests' involves some quantification of the balance of burden versus benefits from earlier diagnosis. The problem also arises of informed consent and who should decide whether screening is appropriate. Parents are responsible for their child's health and they have not only the right but the duty to make good medical decisions on their child's behalf. Earlier diagnosis will confer benefit if earlier detection and intervention improves overall prognosis and/or quality of life. The identification of such children allows the initiation of appropriate preventative or surveillance programmes. However, there are significant concerns about labelling a child as having a cancer predisposition:

1. *The genetic heterogeneity of cancer predisposition.* Disease penetrance (whether individuals carrying susceptibility gene mutations will actually develop disease) varies significantly, e.g. 90% of children with genes for hereditary retinoblastoma and FAP will develop cancer, whereas for Li-Fraumeni penetrance is lower.
2. *The technical problems of testing.* False-positive and false-negative results lead to unnecessary (and often invasive) investigation and false reassurance, respectively. Testing is also expensive.
3. *Psychological/emotional issues.* Coming to terms with the possibility of future cancer development can have enormous impact on the child and family and on family dynamics. The possibiltiy of 'genetic discrimination' may also reduce the chance of acceptance for life insurance and alter job prospects.

The concept of *the rule of earliest onset* would seem a logical starting point in deciding which children should be screened. This states that genetic testing should be permitted no earlier than the age of first possible onset of cancer. Using FAP as an example, an autosomal dominant condition associated with mutation in the adenomatosis polyposis coli gene on chromosome 5, because most affected individuals can expect to have colorectal cancer before the age of 40, but from as young as 10 years of age, and because of the significant risk of cancer in these children, yearly colonoscopy is recommended from the age of 10 years. A positive genetic test would confirm the requirement for this and subsequent 'prophylactic' colectomy. However, a negative test would spare the child from annual colonoscopic surveillance. The success of this approach relies on the high penetrance of the disease with this genetic mutation.

REFERENCES
Kodish E D 1999 Testing children for cancer genes: the rule of earliest onset. J Pediatr 135: 390–395

Oncology, haematology, and rheumatology

Nichols K E, Li F P, Haber D A, Diller L 1998 Childhood cancer predisposition: applications of molecular testing and future implications. J Pediatr 132: 389–397

Quesnel S, Malkin D 1998 Genetic predisposition to cancer and familial cancer syndromes. Pediatr Clin N Am 44: 791–808

Rubnitz J E, Crist W M 1997 Molecular genetics of childhood cancer: implications for pathogenesis, diagnosis, and treatment. Pediatrics 100: 101–108

COMPLICATIONS OF CHEMOTHERAPY AND RADIOTHERAPY

Q. What are the problems associated with chemotherapy and radiotherapy in the treatment of childhood cancers?

To address this question adequately I will divide my answer into four broad sections:

— general side-effects of chemotherapeutic agents
— specific and idiosyncratic side-effects of individual drugs
— long-term sequelae of chemotherapy
— side-effects of radiotherapy

General side-effects of chemotherapy

The majority of childhood cancers today are treated with nationally-coordinated, intensive, combination – chemotherapy/radiotherapy protocols that are greatly improving long-term remission rates. The non-selective mechanisms of action and resulting low therapeutic indices of the anti-cancer drugs mean, however, that a high incidence of potentially severe toxicity must be tolerated in order to administer effective doses of these agents. In particular, those systems with rapidly proliferating cells (bone marrow, gastrointestinal tract, hair follicles) commonly demonstrate toxicity (myelosuppression, nausea and vomiting, oro-intestinal mucositis, and alopecia). The severity of these side-effects depends on the dose and frequency of administration, and the recovery time allowed between treatment courses.

Almost all agents cause nausea and vomiting, marrow suppression (bleomycin being an exception, but it is rarely used in childhood), alopecia and stomatitis. Very often it is *nausea and vomiting* that is most feared by children having chemotherapy. It is therefore imperative that anti-emetic agents are started in anticipation of problems and continued throughout the period of rapid cell turnover. Medications used include metoclopramide, lorazepam, nabilone (a synthetic cannabinoid) and ondansetron (a selective 5-HT$_3$-receptor antagonist, used extensively in paediatric oncology because of its efficacy and minimal side-effects).

At presentation, children with cancer may be neutropenic, anaemic and thrombocytopenic due to bone marrow involvement. Virtually all agents used will result in further damage to the stem cells. The resulting *neutropenia and thrombocytopenia* are the main problems and may lead to their own potentially fatal sequelae.

Alopecia is a distressing side-effect of treatment, particularly for the older child. If dealt with appropriately and sensitively it should cause little problem to the patient or family.

Specific side-effects of chemotherapy

a) *Cardiotoxicity* — most notably cardiotoxic are the anthracyclines, doxorubicin and daunorubicin. This frequently fatal dose-related side-effect has no treatment other than transplantation and is difficult to detect (except by endomyocardial biopsy) until permanent damage has occurred. Monitoring with echocardiography is advised.

b) *Pulmonary toxicity* — bleomycin is the major culprit, with lung damage occurring in 10% of patients and death in 1–2%. Again, damage is dose-related.

c) *Neurotoxicity* — vincristine, an alkaloid agent, most commonly produces a mixed distal sensorimotor neuropathy with long-term use. Initial sensory changes with paraesthesia progress to loss of deep tendon reflexes, an indication to stop the drug as severe incoordination and seizures may develop. Vincristine also causes autonomic dysfunction, commonly resulting in troublesome constipation.

d) *Urological toxicity* — many cytotoxic agents are excreted by the kidneys and it is therefore important to check renal function prior to initiating a course of chemotherapy. Pre- , peri- and post-hydration plus alkalinisation of the urine can prevent or minimise cytotoxic deposition and consequent damage to the renal tubules. Methotrexate, cisplatin, ifosphamide, and carboplatin are all potentially nephrotoxic. *Dose adjustment in renal impairment is mandatory.*

The alkylating agents cyclophosphamide and ifosphamide can cause haemorrhagic cystitis, having a cumulative and dose-related effect. Acrolein, one of the breakdown products of these agents, is the causative substance. Adequate hydration and mesna administration lessens this damage.

I have mentioned only the more common and well-known side-effects of agents used widely in paediatric oncology. However, the agents can have an effect on other systems, including skin, bones and joints, electrolyte balance, liver, etc. and each agent can affect more than one system, for example cyclophosphamide can cause sterility, cardio- and pulmonary toxicity.

Long-term effects of chemotherapy

With over 60% of children treated for cancer now achieving long-term survival (compared with 29% 5-year survival in 1955), long-term side-effects take on heightened importance.

For children who relapse or who are on prolonged chemotherapy courses, there will be long periods of time in hospital and concomitant time away from siblings, peers, friends and, very importantly, school. During this time the whole dynamics of the family may change considerably, ranging from engendering stability as the family rallies round in support, to complete disruption if one or other family member is unable to cope with the inevitable change in lifestyle. Sibling rivalry may cause a great deal of antagonism as another child loses the once equal share of parental attention. Financially, the family may be disadvantaged because of frequent travel between home and hospital, and because one or both parents may have to give up their employment to take up the full time job of looking after their child.

The long-term sequelae of chemotherapy that can be difficult to broach with the patient include:

a) *Infertility* — more a problem for boys than for girls and compounded by radiotherapy. In adolescents and young adults, sperm cryopreservation is justifiable.
b) *Late recurrence* — after a 5-year long-term remission most would be considered 'cured' of the cancer, but relapse can occur after this time.
c) *Secondary neoplasia* — occurs in between 1 and 4% of childhood patients. The increased risk is dependent upon the nature of the cancer, the chemotherapy used, and whether or not radiotherapy was given.

Radiotherapy side-effects

Irradiation, irrespective of age, target site, and total exposure dose can cause acute skin burns.

There are several factors that dictate other possible or likely side-effects:

1. The *total dose* of radiation. A protracted low-dose regime to minimise acute effects may lead to unacceptable late complications.
2. *Timing*. Irradiation exposure prior to full development of tissues can lead to failure of normal development, e.g. irradiation to epiphyseal growth plates can lead to premature closure and asymmetrical limb length in adult life.
3. *Site* of irradiation

   — chest — heart failure
   — cranial — 'somnolence syndrome' (lethargy, irritability, seen in 50% of children 4–8 weeks after treatment); intellectual impairment (particularly in the younger children); short stature ($\downarrow$ growth hormone secretion)
   — neck — hypothyroidism
   — gonads — infertility

Radiation-induced secondary cancers are seen, mostly being soft tissue sarcomas, breast, skin, brain and thyroid cancers.

Tips

● In the heat of the moment it is virtually impossible to recall the specific side-effects of individual chemotherapeutic agents. However, we all remember the endless admissions to the oncology wards with febrile neutropenia, ordering platelets by the gallon for thrombocytopenia, and prescribing bucketfuls of ondansetron for emesis. This is a good starting point.

● Wherever possible, try to break the question down into subheadings. This not only demonstrates an organised thinking pattern, but prevents you from rushing in with the first thing that springs to mind (that could get you taking the first shovel of earth from the hole you are about to dig yourself!)

MEDICAL ASPECTS OF SPLENECTOMY

Q. What advice would you give to a child (and their parents) who has had a splenectomy?

The major long-term risk after splenectomy, or for children with functional hyposplenism, is fulminant life-threatening infection. Splenic macrophages play a significant role in filtering and phagocytosis of bacteria from the circulation and the spleen produces significant amounts of antibody. Without this, overwhelming postsplenectomy infection (OPSI) is a lifelong risk, particularly from encapsulated organisms such as *Streptococcus pneumoniae*. Other common organisms include *Haemophilus influenzae* B, meningococcus, and group A streptococci. My postsplenectomy advice is also pertinent to those children with *congenital aplasia of the spleen* and those with *functional hypoplasia* (as in sickle cell disease, thalassaemia, coeliac disease, ulcerative colitis, rheumatoid arthritis and others).

Ideally, at least 14 days prior to splenectomy (or as soon as possible afterwards) children should be *vaccinated* against pneumococcal, meningococcal and Hib infections. Booster injections with pneumococcal vaccine should be considered every 5–6 years, although there is no evidence-based research that I am aware of to back this up. I would also offer annual influenza immunisation, although good evidence of benefit for this is also lacking.

All patients should be commenced on *chemoprophylaxis* and remain on it for life. Traditionally, penicillin has been the drug of choice, although erythromycin and Augmentin are suitable alternatives. Despite vaccination and prophylactic antibiotics, children and adults are still at increased risk of overwhelming bacterial infection. Any person who has been rendered asplenic and who presents with rigors, pyrexia and malaise of unknown cause should be hospitalised and given intravenous antibiotics.

Failure of chemoprophylaxis may occur because of the development of penicillin-resistant pneumococci. Unfortunately, these organisms may also be resistant to third-generation cephalosporins and so if there is any doubt in a febrile, unwell patient, vancomycin should be added to the intravenous therapy until sensitivities are known.

Besides immuno- and chemo-prophylaxis for 'splenectomised' patients, *education* must be a part of the overall care. Patients should wear a 'Medicalert' bracelet and they should be advised to seek prompt medical attention if unwell. All healthcare professionals involved, including dentists, should be informed of the patient's splenic status.

There is a lack of consensus as to whether chemoprophylaxis is necessary for 2 years, 5 years, until adulthood, or for life, following splenectomy. There are, however, isolated case reports of OPSI occurring decades after splenectomy and so I would recommend prophylaxis for life, despite the risk of developing antimicrobial resistance.

REFERENCE

Brigden M L, Pattullo A L 1999 Prevention and management of overwhelming postsplenectomy infection — an update. Crit Care Med 27: 836–842

Oncology, haematology, and rheumatology

BONE MARROW TRANSPLANTATION

Q. What do you know about bone marrow transplantation in children?

Bone marrow transplantation (BMT) involves the harvesting and transfer of stem cells from a donor to a recipient. The transplanted cells may be from the individual themselves (*autologous*); from a genetically different person (*allogenic*); or from an identical twin (*synergenic*). There are numerous *indications* for bone marrow transplantation in children but these can be divided into three main categories:

1. Replacement of absent or non-functioning cells, e.g. of immunodeficiencies (SCID); red cells (thalassaemia); myeloid cells (primary neutropenias); or of all cell types (aplastic anaemia, marrow hypoplasia due to chemotherapy).
2. Generation of a specific lymphoid cell-mediated action in the host, e.g. graft-versus-leukaemia effect (malignant disease, ALL, AML).
3. Generation of cells that are able to produce missing enzymes in the host, e.g. mucopolysaccharidoses.

Allogenic transplantations usually come from human leukocyte antigen-(HLA) identical siblings or from matched unrelated donors (MUD). However, as only 25% of siblings are compatible, the number of MUDs used is increasing. A good HLA match is essential for good graft survival. The major disadvantage of allogenic transplantation is graft versus host disease.

In *autologous transplantations*, the patient receives her own marrow or peripheral stem cells so HLA matching is not needed and there is no graft-versus-host disease. However, there is an increased risk of disease relapse due to undetected cancer cells in the autologous marrow. In an attempt to reduce this, neoplastic cells are removed from the harvested marrow (purging), using chemotherapy and monoclonal antibodies.

Q. OK, I'll stop you there. Outline the stages a child undergoing a BMT would go through.

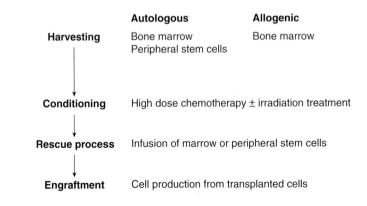

	Autologous	Allogenic
Harvesting	Bone marrow Peripheral stem cells	Bone marrow
Conditioning	High dose chemotherapy ± irradiation treatment	
Rescue process	Infusion of marrow or peripheral stem cells	
Engraftment	Cell production from transplanted cells	

Post transplantation management involves the prevention and management of the side-effects of high-dose chemotherapy ± irradiation. Barrier nursing is essential to avoid infection as children are severely immunocompromised. Haematopoietic growth factors are used to enhance engraftment. Patients are treated with blood products, antibiotics, antivirals and antifungals as required.

Q. You mentioned graft versus host disease. Explain what you understand by this term.

Graft-versus-host disease (GVHD) is a potentially serious complication seen in allogenic bone marrow transplantation, occurring because transplanted T cells in the graft attack the host. If it occurs within 3 months of transplantation, it is called acute GVHD, and at any time after that, chronic GVHD. Acute GVHD is classically characterised by skin rash, hepatitis and jaundice. The risk of GVHD is reduced by T-cell depletion of grafts using monoclonal antibodies. After transplantation, patients are routinely given immunosuppressive drugs such as cyclosporin to suppress T cells.

REFERENCE
Stanworth S J 1998 Bone marrow transplantation in children. Curr Paediatr 8: 78–82

Oncology, haematology, and rheumatology

MANAGEMENT OF NEUTROPENIA

Q. How would you manage a leukaemic child with chemotherapy–induced neutropenia?

Neutropenia in children with leukaemia may be secondary to bone marrow infiltration or bone marrow suppression by cytotoxic drugs. The child is at risk from bacterial and fungal infection when the neutrophil count is $<1.0\times10^9$/L. Life-threatening infections are more likely to occur at neutrophil counts of $<0.2\times10^9$/L. It should be remembered that these children also have secondary lymphopenia and impaired immunoglobulin production.

The timing of chemotherapy-induced neutropenia can usually be predicted and preventative measures should be taken. Neutropenia itself does not require treatment but it is essential to avoid unnecessary infection. The pathogens that most frequently cause infection are the patient's own normal flora: skin flora, such as *Staphylococcus aureus* and *Staphylococcus epidermis*; and bowel flora, such as coliforms, *Pseudomonas* and *Klebsiella*.

Systemic infection by organisms that are normal commensals in the mouth can be reduced by using mouthwashes such as 0.1% Hibitane. If mouth ulcers develop, Difflam can be used with great success as it is both antibacterial and has local anaesthetic properties. *Candida* infection of the mucous membranes can be reduced by the regular use of an oral antifungal drug such as nystatin. Nystatin is not absorbed and therefore has no role in systemic infection. For those at particularly high risk of fungal infection, for example after bone marrow transplantation, an oral drug such as ketoconazole or fluconazole might be more effective. It is important that children avoid vigorous teeth brushing as this may introduce bacteria into the bloodstream.

Neutropenic children are at great risk of *iatrogenic infection* and for this reason handwashing by staff and relatives must be meticulous. This is especially important when taking blood, especially from central venous lines, when a strict aseptic technique must be used. Rectal examination and the administration of drugs per rectum must be avoided as the rectal mucosa is thin and easily damaged, allowing entry of Gram-negative organisms into the bloodstream.

As mentioned earlier, children with neutropenia alone do not require treatment. However, any neutropenic child who is unwell with non-specific symptoms, or is peripherally shut down, or has a fever of 38°C on more than two separate occasions in a 12-hour period should be screened for infection. This should include surface and throat swabs, and blood and urine cultures. Swabs from the entry site and central blood cultures must be done in all children with a central venous line. Broad-spectrum antibiotics must be started immediately, without waiting for culture results. In the unit that I work in, the first-line antibiotics used are piperacillin and tobramycin. If the temperature has not settled at 72 hours then the patient is changed to second-line antibiotics, imipenem and tobramycin. If the patient is still pyrexial after a further 48 hours then I would be suspicious of a systemic fungal infection and would introduce amphotericin B. Amphotericin should be given initially as a small test-dose and it is important to monitor electrolytes as hypokalaemia is commonly seen. If the blood cultures are negative, antibiotics are given for a minimum of 5 days providing the child has been apyrexial for 48 hours. If the blood cultures are positive, antibiotics are adjusted accordingly and given for a minimum course of 7 days.

JUVENILE CHRONIC ARTHRITIS

Q. How would you assess an 8-year-old girl presenting with a 4-month history of joint pain?

Firstly, I would want to find out more about the nature of the illness. I would ask which joints were affected by pain and whether there was any associated joint swelling, warmth, or restricted movement. I would ask whether there had been any obvious triggering illness as the arthritis might be reactive, following a viral infection. I would also ask whether the child had been systemically unwell at the time of onset of joint pain, taking note of the presence of a generalised macular rash suggestive of systemic juvenile chronic arthritis, although this is more common in the younger child.

I would do a careful examination, ensuring that I did not hurt the child. I would examine each joint for the presence of swelling, warmth, erythema, tenderness, and range of movement. I would look for signs of muscle-wasting around each joint, suggesting chronic disuse. The number and type (i.e. large or small) of joints affected is used to classify juvenile chronic arthritis into oligoarthritis, polyarthritis, or systemic arthritis on clinical findings. I would check for a rash, lymphadenopathy, and hepatosplenomegaly, although these are usually found at the onset of disease in systemic arthritis. I would also look for a scaly skin rash and nail pitting in the patient and close relatives, as psoriasis can be associated with an aggressive form of chronic arthritis.

There is no diagnostic test for arthritis and most of the assessment is done on clinical grounds. However, I would arrange a full blood count, which might show anaemia and thrombocytosis, and ESR, which will confirm the current state of inflammation. I would check for rheumatoid factor, which is negative in the majority of cases, and antinuclear factor. (In an older boy, I would also check for human leukocyte antigen B27, which tends to be associated with lower limb arthritides and is related to adult ankylosing spondylitis.)

I would arrange for an ophthalmologist to examine this girl, looking for signs of iridocyclitis, which can be associated with antinuclear factor-positive chronic arthritis in young girls, leading to visual impairment.

Q. So, how would you manage the girl once you have made the diagnosis of juvenile chronic arthritis?

The main aims of my management would be good pain relief and rehabilitation. In terms of pain relief, I would start with *non-steroidal anti-inflammatory drugs (NSAIDs)*, such as ibuprofen or naproxen. I tend to use these two as I am most familiar with their side-effect profile. This includes abdominal pain, caused by gastritis (and even ulceration) and, rarely, interstitial nephritis. I would use NSAIDs cautiously in a child with asthma, as they might cause an exacerbation of symptoms.

NSAIDs have analgesic and antipyretic effects in addition to the anti-inflammatory effect. Their main action is to inhibit cyclo-oxygenase activity, thereby reducing prostaglandin synthesis. These may need to be given in quite high doses. It may be necessary to change from one drug to another if there is no improvement after several weeks, as some children will respond to one better than to another. It may be necessary to use *physical therapies* for pain relief, particularly joint splints, in the acute stages of inflammation. These are also used to maintain joint position and avoid the development of contractures.

Children usually respond well to NSAIDs but it is sometimes necessary to use *second-line agents*, such as methotrexate or cyclosporin A if there is no improvement. These are used in low dosage, but I would be reluctant to start them without expert advice as they have serious side-effects.

Juvenile chronic arthritis can cause impaired function of joints, leading to severe physical disability. The aim of *rehabilitation* with physiotherapy and occupational therapy is to avoid fixed deformity. Both therapists should be involved from an early stage and will need the full cooperation of the whole family, since the exercise regime is likely to be arduous. Once pain relief is achieved, an exercise regime will be developed which maintains joint mobility and muscular strength. This may include the use of a hydrotherapy pool, as swimming is good exercise in which the joints are fully supported.

As with any chronic illness, I would want to be certain that the child was getting adequate *nutrition*. Children with juvenile chronic arthritis are often tired and uncomfortable and their appetite may be poor as a result. High-calorie foods should be encouraged. I would also ensure that the child was fully integrated at school as soon as possible, both for educational and social purposes.

REFERENCE

Schneider R, Laxer R M 1998 Systemic-onset juvenile rheumatoid arthritis. Baillières Clin Rheumatol 12: 245–271

LYMPHADENOPATHY

Q. How would you approach the problem of a child referred with lymphadenopathy?

My priority would be to exclude serious causes of lymphadenopathy, such as *acute leukaemia*. I would start by taking a history, particularly looking for a recent history of weight loss, lethargy, bruising, or bleeding. I would check for pallor, bruising, petechiae, and hepatosplenomegaly on examination. If my findings suggested acute leukaemia, I would urgently check a full blood count and film and consider arranging a bone marrow aspiration. If the lump was hard, enlarging, or tethered, or associated with other lymphadenopathy or hepatosplenomegaly, I would consider *lymphoma* as a cause. I would arrange for a chest X-ray and possibly chest and abdominal CT scans. Biopsy of the node would be necessary to make a definitive diagnosis.

Another cause of lymphadenopathy, which is important to exclude urgently, is *Kawasaki disease*. The diagnosis is made on clinical signs and I would expect to find a miserable child with a history of at least 5 days of swinging pyrexia associated with cervical lymph nodes, bilateral non-purulent conjunctivitis, a swollen red tongue or lips, a generalised maculopapular rash, or oedematous extremities. At a later stage, there might be peeling of the hands and feet. Many of these symptoms are non-specific, but if four of these features were found in addition to the swinging pyrexia, I would treat the child for Kawasaki disease, as the consequences of not treating include ischaemic heart disease. I would start high-dose aspirin and give intravenous immunoglobulins, while arranging for an ECG and echocardiogram, which might reveal coronary artery dilatation (see page 125).

It is more usual to be faced with a child who is not particularly unwell, but has a history of lymphadenopathy, often associated with symptoms suggestive of a viral infection, such as a sore throat, fever, or a generalised rash. It may be possible to establish the identity of the particular virus if the lymphadenopathy is associated with a distinctive rash (for example, the generalised morbilliform rash of *measles*, which classically starts behind the ears after a prodromal illness). However, measles and rubella are less commonly seen since immunisation programmes have included them and it is more usual to see lymphadenopathy in children with non-specific illness due to glandular fever, cytomegalovirus or toxoplasmosis infection. There may be no clinical features specifically suggestive of *glandular fever* (caused by the Epstein Barr virus), but it tends to affect teenagers and may be associated with hepatosplenomegaly and prolonged malaise. Blood film usually reveals atypical mononuclear cells and a test based on finding agglutinins may give a rapid diagnosis. It is possible to look at viral titres, preferably specific EBV IgM antibodies, as these will suggest *recent* infection if present. *Cytomegalovirus* may demonstrate very similar clinical features to glandular fever and can be diagnosed by detection of inclusion bodies in fresh urine samples. *Toxoplasmosis* is a protozoal infection which may give a similar clinical picture, with persistent lymphadenopathy. Positive antibody titres may be reassuring to the family.

I would consider *bacterial infection* if the child had localised lymph-adenopathy. Glands may become swollen in the region of a staphylococcal infection, for example groin nodes in cellulitis of the leg or in the axilla or neck following immunisations. Cervical glands enlarge with *tonsillitis*. Sometimes, an individual gland develops bacterial infection and may go on to form an abscess. The gland is usually red and very tender. If pus has formed, the lump may fluctuate on palpation. It will require drainage if antibiotics do not reduce the swelling. *Tuberculosis* should be considered if isolated lymph nodes are persistently swollen. There may be a history of tuberculosis in the family, or a family member with a chronic cough. Checking a Mantoux test will make the diagnosis.

Tip

● This is the sort of question you may be asked as an opener. You can approach 'non-urgent' clinical scenarios either by mentioning most common causes first, or by mentioning the conditions that are most important to exclude. Try and give a few distinguishing features (either on history or on examination) rather than a long list.

REFERENCE
Morland B, 1995 Lymphodenopathy. Arch Dis Child 73: 476–479

Miscellaneous

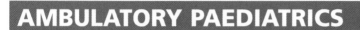

AMBULATORY PAEDIATRICS

Q. Ambulatory paediatrics — what is it, and why do it?

Despite significant reductions in childhood morbidity and mortality over the last few decades, admissions to hospital in the UK have risen dramatically. The majority of children admitted to hospital have mild illness, are admitted for short periods, and require observation rather than treatment. This begs the question, 'Does the child need admission at all?' and has given rise to the concept (or philosophy) of ambulatory paediatrics. As long ago as 1976 the Court report advised that, 'whenever the illness and circumstances allow, a child will be cared for at home'. Ambulatory paediatrics essentially incorporates this concept with the desire to reduce hospital admissions. A number of services can be employed to prevent hospital admission or expedite hospital discharge. These include:

— telephone hotlines for GPs
— out-of-hours telephone access for parents — 'NHS Direct'
— outreach clinics
— 'rapid-response' clinics
— day assessment/observation wards
— paediatric community nurse services

Audit has shown that the majority of children seen acutely in hospital are seen out-of-hours (6 p.m. to 8 a.m.). Generally speaking, this is the time that the most inexperienced paediatricians (or A&E staff) are working unsupervised. Maximising the efficiency of services during the day may therefore have little impact on reducing hospital admissions unless these services extend beyond the normal working day. Detractors of ambulatory paediatrics argue this point, stating that what is required is to have a consultant-led service with consultants on the 'shop floor' at all hours of the day and night!

Having said that, there is evidence to suggest that the measures above do improve the service and reduce hospital admissions. Medical queries from GPs or parents may sometimes be dealt with effectively over the phone. Some hospitals have adopted a 1-hour period in the day when GPs are able to phone the on-call consultant of the day, for example 11 a.m to 12 noon. This could coincide with the consultant's rapid-response clinic for urgent, but not acute, referrals. Parents may have anxieties about their child that can be dealt with by phone, although there are legal implications of unrecorded telephone advice. I am unaware of parental hotlines to consultants in paediatrics but the government has set up phone helplines to nurse practitioners (NHS Direct).

Over 50% of admissions to hospital are with minor illnesses, including breathing difficulties, fits, and fever. Provided the right social set-up is in place, these children may be better managed at home after a short period of observation and/or treatment to ensure that there is no further deterioration. Good examples of this are children with a febrile convulsion or croup. Many hospitals now have observation wards running from 8 a.m. to late evening. Any child that, clinically or socially, cannot be managed at home by 'closing time' can then be admitted to the ward overnight. Consultant-led ward rounds in the late evening ensure experienced decision-making.

Perhaps the greatest improvement in the service has been the introduction of *paediatric community nurses*. These highly skilled nurses are hospital-based but work in the community. Not only can they provide excellent follow-up (either by telephone or face to face) for children with acute illness but they also provide the means for keeping children with chronic disease out of hospital. Where, previously, children would require prolonged hospital admission they can now be managed at home. Examples of this include children with fractured femurs on traction, children with cystic fibrosis requiring three-monthly courses of intravenous antibiotics, and nasogastrically fed neonates.

Although the philosophy of keeping children out of hospital is not new, ambulatory paediatrics and the approaches mentioned above are still in their infancy. Hospitals are moving towards this approach more and more. Its effectiveness (or not) will become apparent with time and audit.

Tips

● This is a hot topic. Something has to be done to alleviate the chronic bed shortages seen in paediatrics, particularly over winter. The examiner may be fishing for innovative ways of solving the problem in his hospital. Come up with a way of halving hospital admissions and you are guaranteed to pass!

● The political tide is moving towards consultants providing a greater out-of-hours service and being resident on-call in the future. You just may be asked if you would consider taking up a post as a resident (or junior) consultant after 5 years of Calman training. There is no right or wrong answer to this question — you are on your own with this one!

● Audit is always a favourite with the examiners. Introduce the subject, as we have done, at the end if you are knowledgeable on the subject, especially if you have undertaken a useful piece of audit in the past.

● The effectiveness of NHS Direct in reducing the burden on GP and hospital services is not clear as yet. However, testing the system with hypothetical clinical problems has demonstrated significant disparity in the advice given. The service may, in fact, have *increased* the burden on primary practice as patients and parents seek further medical advice following telephone discussion. Further studies are required before it can be declared an overwhelming success or a very expensive 'white elephant'!

REFERENCES

Beverley D W, Ball R J, Smith R A et al 1997 Planning for the future: the experience of implementing a children's day assessment unit in a district general hospital. Arch Dis Child 77: 287–293

Committee on child health services 1976 Court report. Fit for the future. HMSO, London

MacFaul R, Stewart M, Werneke U et al 1998 Parental and professional perception of need for emergency admission to hospital: prospective questionnaire-based study. Arch Dis Child 79: 213–218

Meates M 1997 Ambulatory paediatrics — making a difference. Arch Dis Child 76: 468–476

Munro J, Nicholl J, O'Cathain A et al 2000 Impact of NHS Direct on demand for immediate care: observational study. Br Med J 321: 150–153

Stewart M, Werneke U, MacFaul R et al 1998 Medical and social factors associated with the admission and discharge of acutely ill children. Arch Dis Child 79: 219–224

PASS ✓

Miscellaneous

EVIDENCE-BASED MEDICINE

Q. What do you understand by the term 'evidence-based medicine'?

Evidence-based medicine is a term used to describe the use of current best available evidence in making decisions about the clinical care of an individual patient. Of course, this is not a new concept and physicians have been aiming to base their clinical decisions on scientific evidence for many years, albeit not necessarily in a structured manner. However, it is true to say that sometimes evidence has taken some considerable time to be applied in clinical medicine (for example the use of antenatal corticosteroids in women in preterm labour).

The term 'evidence-based medicine' means more than applying the findings from a single research paper to your patient. Firstly, you need to find *high quality evidence related to a particular clinical question*. It is important that the clinician identifies exactly what is important to know. For example, when faced with a child with croup, the paediatrician needs to decide precisely which therapeutic issue needs to be resolved. Is it simply whether steroids are useful in croup; is it which form of corticosteroid is most effective; is it which is the most cost-effective preparation to use; or is it which is most likely to reduce the length of hospital stay?

Once the question is formulated, it is important to think of some search terms in order to minimise 'missed' research. I would therefore think of alternative terms for croup (such as laryngotracheitis and stridor) and alternative terms for steroids (such as corticosteroids, dexamethasone and budesonide). I would put these search terms into a database such as Medline, and see how many 'hits' I found. If there were a lot of hits, I would narrow the search down further by adding in an outcome, such as mortality, admission to intensive care units, or total length of hospital stay. For ordinary clinical use, this sort of basic search should come up with some research papers appropriate to my patient.

When doing a more thorough search, it is important to consider *possible sources of bias*. It is easy to ignore papers published in foreign languages, but these should be translated and included. I usually put my search strategy through two databases, for example Embase, in order to include more European papers. It is also important to avoid dismissing papers published in less well-known journals. They should be assessed on the same criteria as those published in the *Lancet*. Unfortunately, many papers showing a negative outcome are not published. This is a difficult bias to avoid and obviously has great influence on the outcome of your search. Some of these papers may be published on 'grey' databases, for example if they were written up as an MD thesis, and these should be assessed for completeness.

It can be difficult to find good quality research addressing the most frequently asked questions in paediatrics. For example, many drugs have not been thoroughly tested for use in children.

Once I had obtained details of relevant research papers, I would critically appraise them. Ideally, I would look at a meta-analysis or systematic review addressing my clinical question, but if none were available, I would analyse all of the randomised controlled trials. It is sometimes possible to find summaries of evidence, for example in the Cochrane Database.

Q. So, what is the Cochrane Database?

The Cochrane Database is a collection of systematic reviews, which can be obtained via the Internet or on CD ROM. Articles are published by members of the Cochrane Collaboration, who apply a strict set of criteria to research studies after thorough searching for appropriate scientific papers. As yet, there are not many Cochrane Reviews which apply to the paediatric population, but numbers are increasing and certain groups, such as the neonatology group, have published a large number of appraisals of research studies.

A disadvantage of using the database may be that the questions addressed tend to be broad-based and may not necessarily apply to your individual patient. In this case, the original articles can be obtained so that you can appraise them yourself.

Q. Is this how NICE makes its decisions?

The National Institute of Clinical Excellence (NICE) has been established in order to assess the evidence on the use of certain therapies in clinical conditions. I assume that the Institute will use similar methodology in their assessments, but I am not aware whether they use the Cochrane summaries or appraise individual research papers themselves.

The aim is to ensure that patients receive the same care nationally, according to guidelines and recommendations, where there is good evidence of clinical effectiveness, rather than as a result of the decision of an individual physician. As yet, I am unaware of any treatments used in paediatrics that have undergone this process. (A well-known example of a drug studied by NICE is Viagra, used in erectile dysfunction.)

One of the difficulties with such national guidelines is that the evidence may not apply to an individual patient, for example where poor compliance with complicated treatment regimes may be an issue. The Institute may only be able to offer broad advice and will need to continually update their guidelines as newer evidence emerges.

REFERENCE
Christakis D A, Davis R, Rivara F P 2000 Pediatric evidence-based medicine: past, present and future. J Pediatr 136: 383–389

DESIGNING A RESEARCH STUDY

Q. From your reading of the literature, what different forms do you think medical research can take?

The most powerful and convincing research takes the form of projects organised to analyse specific problems. These often have a statistical basis and may be *observational* (e.g. case-control or cohort studies) or *experimental* (e.g. clinical trials). *Case reports* and *clinical observations* do not strictly fall into the framework of statistical studies in medicine. They are, however, a valuable source of medical information despite their anecdotal nature.

Q. What are the main distinguishing features of medical studies?

The major classification of medical studies is into longitudinal or cross-sectional studies. *Longitudinal* studies investigate a process over a defined period of time and observations are made on more than one occasion — examples are clinical trials and cohort studies. *Cross-sectional* studies analyse a phenomenon fixed in time and involve only one observation.

Studies may also be prospective or retrospective. In *prospective* studies, data is collected forwards in time from the start of the study. In *retrospective* studies data is collected from past events and may, for example, be collected from patients' notes. Studies may also be *randomised* or *non-randomised*.

Q. What do you understand by the term 'clinical trial'?

A clinical trial is defined as a prospective study which examines the relative efficacy of interventions such as drug treatments in *human* subjects. In most situations, this involves comparing standard treatment (the control group) with new therapy (the experimental group).

Q. What do you know about the organisation of drug trials?

Trials in the pharmaceutical industry are divided into four phases:

Phase 1   Clinical pharmacology and toxicology studies
— involves healthy volunteers
— pharmacokinetic studies (absorption, distribution, metabolism, excretion)
— pharmacodynamic studies
Phase 2   Clinical investigation
— patients
— pharmacokinetics, pharmacodynamics
— dose-ranging studies

Phase 3 Evaluation of treatment
— randomised controlled trials
— comparison with other drugs
Phase 4 Post-marketing studies
— further safety and efficacy surveillance studies

Q. Tell me how you would go about designing a clinical research study.

Effective clinical research needs careful planning. When organising a research study, I would always contact the local research and development (R&D) department for help from an early stage. I would organise my study around the following points:

1. *Define the research question*: refine and focus research *ideas* into research *questions* to be answered.
2. *Search of the literature*:
   — has the study been done before?
   — ideas for research design
   — Medline / Pubmed
3. *Study design*: i.e. type of study
   — drug, dose, age group, time period, longitudinal, randomisation, double-blind, placebo, multicentre, statistician input.
4. *Planning*:
   — study
   — achievable aims, time available, suitable study population, recruitment, outcome measurements
   — statistics
   — numbers needed, power calculation, length of study to achieve numbers
5. *Supervision*:
   — who to approach for support, guidance, advice, expertise?
   — who to involve if forming a study *group*?
6. *Funding*:
   — apply for research grant
   — list of possible funding from local R&D, support from pharmaceutical company
   — estimate money required
   — salary, consumables, research nurse
7. *Ethics*: contact local ethics committee — approval will be needed.
8. *Information leaflets*: prepare parental/child information leaflets.
9. *Pilot study*: will this be needed?
10. *Analyse results of pilot study*: ? alter study design.
11. *Study period*.
12. *Analyse results*.

Q. You mentioned power calculations — tell me a little more about them.

Power calculations are used to calculate the appropriate sample size for a clinical trial. Most good studies have a power of 80–90%. It is important to use power calculations before starting the trial to calculate required sample sizes, so ensuring that any difference seen is statistically significant.

Q. Tell me a little more about randomisation.

Randomisation is a procedure in which chance determines the assignment of a subject to the alternative groups under investigation. Randomisation produces study groups that are comparable for the unknown, hidden attributes as well as the known attributes, which may influence the outcome in addition to the treatment itself. Randomisation therefore *avoids bias*.

The process of randomisation may be simple, such as tossing a coin to allocate patients, or may be more complex, involving random number charts or computer programmes.

Single-blind randomisation is when the patient and parents do not know what treatment is being received. *Double-blind randomisation* is when neither the patient and parents, nor the doctor looking after the patient and assessing the disease process, are aware what treatment is being received.

Stratification is often incorporated within randomisation. For example, you may want to ensure that an equal number of boys and girls are recruited from each centre in a multicentre study — stratification would be used to prevent all the boys being randomly selected from one centre and all the girls from another (the higher the number recruited into the study, the less likely this is to happen by chance).

In *cross-over studies*, patients are given both the drug on trial and the placebo. Randomisation is used to decide the order in which the drugs are given. A *wash-out* period is often included in these studies to avoid the effects of one drug being carried over into the second period.

THE INTERNET

Q. What is your experience of using the Internet for work purposes?

I have found many applications for the Internet in recent years, particularly *medical databases*, when searching for information about a clinical problem. For example, if I see a patient on the ward suffering from severe abdominal pain in association with Henoch-Schönlein purpura, I can search the databases using Medline for papers describing or assessing therapeutic options, for example looking at the use of corticosteroids. When successful therapies can be found which have not yet reached the textbooks, it might make a considerable difference to an individual patient.

Many *journals* now have their papers published on the Net at the same time as they are sent out in printed form. This means that when you are looking for a particular study it may be possible to read it through on-line, rather than going to the library or trying to assess the quality of the paper from an abstract in a medical database.

Information from the Internet is being accessed with increasing frequency by patients and their families. I have been approached by parents in outpatient clinics with information they have discovered about their child's medical condition. Because anybody can create a website about any subject they choose, people with very little knowledge or evidence can put information about a condition on the Net and it may be necessary to point out invalid information to a family. This can be difficult at times because people tend to believe what they read. It is particularly difficult to reassure parents who have found information outside 'conventional' medicine, because they expect you to be cynical about it. I find it useful in these situations to give parents information that *I* have found on the Net which is more appropriate for their needs. I have also found the Net useful for finding *support groups* that may be of interest to the family.

I use *e-mail* when I am working in conjunction with colleagues on projects such as revision of management guidelines or preparation of scientific papers for publication. This has the advantage of speed when compared to post, as well as saving on paper!

I have used the Internet to find *information about training* in paediatrics, for example, when considering the syllabus of a higher specialty. It is also possible to search for *guidelines issued by specialty groups* (for example, on the management of diabetic ketoacidosis which is published on the Web by the Paediatric Endocrine Subspecialty Group).

I have participated in a *discussion group* on the Net with other trainees, when we considered chosen topics. We have discussed diverse issues, from the future of training posts for paediatric registrars to the introduction of the meningococcus vaccination programme. This is very helpful when trainees are geographically isolated.

TEACHING

Q. Tell me about the different methods of teaching you have experience of.

I have now been on 'both sides of the fence' with teaching and in my experience there are some people who naturally are excellent at teaching and others who obviously do not particularly enjoy it! Different teaching methods include:

— formal lectures
— demonstration
— bedside teaching
— tutorials
— self-directed learning
— problem-solving exercises

Some subjects lend themselves particularly well to certain teaching methods. For example, the insertion of an umbilical arterial catheter in a 500 g 25-week baby cannot be taught effectively by means of a formal lecture. The old adage 'see one, do one, teach one' is very apt for such practical procedures. Depending on the level of competence (and confidence!) of the learner, of course, more than one demonstration and supervision of more than one procedure may be required.

In a *formal lecture* it is presumed that members of the audience are all alike in their personality, level of knowledge and experience, language skills, and ability to digest the information given. The material is structured in a way the lecturer chooses and does not take into account any individual needs. The opportunity for questioning and feedback is limited or unavailable altogether. Not surprisingly, most of the material in a formal lecture is almost instantly forgotten. For these reasons, I am not a proponent of this form of learning.

However, if it is necessary to give a formal lecture, there are certain methods I would employ to promote the learning process. On average people remember about 20% of what they hear, but 50–80% of what they both hear and *see*. Therefore, the use of *visual aids* is very powerful in reinforcing information-gathering. There are certain rules about visual aids that are worth bearing in mind:

1. *Use more than one type of visual aid*, e.g mix video, overheads, slides and demonstrations, but know how to use the technology before commencing the lecture. In other words, know which button to press when!
2. *Keep the information on overheads/slides simple, legible and relevant* to the subject. The audience should not have to spend their time trying to decipher overheads or understand the relevance of a holiday snap to the content of the teaching instead of listening to what is being said.
3. Giving *printouts of the overheads or slides* prior to the start of the lecture provides succinct reinforcement of the lecture content and prevents the participants trying to copy the contents of the slides down instead of listening.

The standard formal lecture for medical students lasts for 1 hour. This is far too long to listen to a monologue and actively digest the information. I would limit the duration of a formal lecture to a maximum of 20 minutes.

Q. Tell me then how you would organise a teaching session.

There is a further adage that is not only appropriate to teaching, but to life in general:

Prior planning and preparation prevent poor performance.

A number of questions need to be asked when planning a teaching session:

1. What is the *objective* of the teaching session? Is it to teach a practical skill, to teach about enzymatic pathways, or to convince an examiner that the student should pass the viva section of the MRCPCH exam? This question will direct you to the most suitable teaching method.
2. Who are the *audience*? Are they all at the same level (very unusual) or of mixed abilities?
3. What *facilities* are available? Is there a lecture theatre, a laboratory, projection equipment, or patients to act as guinea-pigs?
4. *How long* have I got?
5. What *format* will maximise learning potential?
6. Will I get any *feedback* on the effectiveness of the teaching (there is nothing like having a colleague observing or, for the more sensitive teacher, a video recording of events, to give feedback)?

Q. What qualities do you think make a good teacher?

Some people are naturally better than others at imparting knowledge. However, anyone who is teaching others should try to:

— create an atmosphere in which the participants do not feel inhibited or threatened. Remember that cooperation, rather than competition, should be encouraged (although certain specialties within medicine may seem to ignore this maxim!)
— employ methods that encourage participants to learn at their own pace
— remain flexible, allowing for the variety of personalities and levels of understanding within the group
— encourage questioning, discussion and feedback
— use language that is appropriate for the audience
— use experiences of the audience as a basis for learning. For example, get the audience to see a child with failure to thrive before going through the management issues for that clinical problem (provided the teaching session is not for 150 medical students, for the sake of the patient!)
— promote ongoing learning by motivating interest and desire to know more

259

Tips

● We can all remember certain teachers during our medical school and post-graduate experience who insisted on scaring us half to death. Sadly we remember the personality but very little of what they actually were trying to teach us! Hopefully, we have moved forward since then (although you may meet one or two of the old school at the membership examination!).

Q. Why do we need statistics?

At its most basic, statistics is the measurement of chance. In most situations it is impossible to analyse a whole population and we therefore need to analyse a small sample of this population. Statistical analysis reveals the degree of accuracy with which our sample reflects the population as a whole. This will be governed by the size of the sample and the nature of the distribution of the variable.

Statistics can also be used to assess the degree of difference between two groups of variables, for example the morning peak flows of children during the weeks immediately before and after the addition of inhaled salmeterol to their therapy. The averages may appear higher after salmeterol but this apparent improvement may merely have been observed by chance. Statistics can be used to analyse the likelihood that this is the case, so-called *statistical significance testing*. Statistics is also used to ensure that the results of medical research are comparable and can be generalised.

A doctor must have a basic knowledge of statistics before undertaking any kind of research. More importantly, most medical papers will use statistical analysis and it is important that the reader is able to comprehend and critically evaluate the published results and conclusions.

Q. What is the difference between qualitative and quantitative data?

Qualitative data are data to which only a quality (and not an exact number) can be ascribed. This may be *nominal* (if they can be classified by a 'name' alone) such as male or female, dead or alive, or blood group, or *ranked* data (if they can be ordered in some way), such as severity of trauma.

Data to which a certain number can be ascribed are said to be *quantitative*. This may be *discrete* (if only certain discrete values are assumed), such as numbers of children, or *continuous* (assuming any value), such as plasma glucose levels.

Q. What do you understand by the term 'normal distribution'?

The characteristics of the distribution of the possible values of a random variable are analysed by plotting the frequency on the vertical axis against the magnitude of the values on the horizontal axis. The variable is said to follow a *normal* or *Gaussian* distribution if the plot is smooth with a characteristic bell-shape, symmetrical about the mean (i.e. the left- and right-hand halves are mirror images). In addition, in normal distribution the *mean*, *median* and *mode* values are all the same — the central value of the variable.

In practice few, if any, variables in biological populations truly follow a normal distribution, though we often make the assumption that they do.

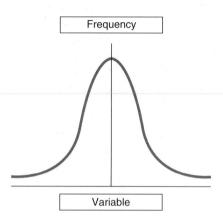

Q. What is binomial distribution?

Data which can only represent a 0 or a 1 response, such as treatment success or failure, are said to follow a binomial distribution.

Q. What are mean, median and mode values?

They are indicators of the central tendency of a distribution. The *mean* is the arithmetic average, i.e. the sum of the values divided by the number of values. The *mode* is the most commonly occurring value. The *median* is the middle value if all the values are placed in rank or ascending order.

Q. What do you understand by the terms 'parametric' and 'non-parametric' tests?

Parametric tests of statistical significance can be used if the variable under consideration follows a normal distribution. An example is the Student's *t*-distribution test, which can be used in two ways. The *paired t-test* is used when paired or matched data are being examined, as in a matched case-control study or a cross-over trial. The *unpaired t-test* is used when the two groups in question are not connected.

    Non-parametric tests are used if the data do not follow a normal distribution. In these situations, the paired *t*-test is replaced by a *Wilcoxon signed rank test*, and the unpaired *t*-test is replaced by the *Wilcoxon test* (also known as the Mann-Whitney *U* test). Non-parametric tests can always be used as no assumptions about the underlying population are made. However, if a near-normal population can be assumed, it is better to use a parametric test as the calculated *P* value will be smaller.

Q. What is the null hypothesis?

The null hypothesis assumes that any apparent difference between two groups of variables has occurred by chance; that, in reality, no difference exists; and that the two groups are really from the same population. The P value is a measure of the probability that the apparent difference has occurred by chance. Different statistical tests can be applied to measure the P value, depending on the nature of the data involved. P values range from 0.00 (0% likelihood that this has occurred by chance) to 1.00 (100% likelihood). We arbitrarily employ a standard of 0.05 and if the P value for the difference in two groups of variables (as calculated by an appropriately chosen statistical test) is less than this (i.e. there is a probability of <0.05, or <5% likelihood, that this difference has occurred by chance), then we reject the null hypothesis. We therefore accept that there is a difference between the two groups and that the two groups of values do not come from the same population.

Q. What do you understand by variance and standard deviation?

The indicators of central tendency such as the mean give no indication of how widely dispersed the measured values of a variable are about the centre. The variance and standard deviation are both measures of scatter of data about the natural mean. The smaller they are, the less the natural scatter.

The *variance* is the average amount by which any individual value (X) differs from the mean ($\bar{X}$) and the *standard deviation* (SD) is the square root of the variance. The standard deviation can easily be used to calculate where values are distributed: 66% of values lie within the range $\bar{X} \pm 1$ SD; 95% of values lie within the range $\bar{X} \pm 2$ SD; 99% of values lie within the range $\bar{X} \pm 3$ SD.

Q. What do you understand by the term 'standard error'?

The standard error is a measure of the uncertainty of a simple statistical parameter. The most commonly quoted is the *standard error of the mean*, which is calculated by dividing the standard deviation by the square root of the number of values in the sample.

Q. What are type I and type II errors?

Significance testing only indicates a balance of probabilities and therefore even conclusions drawn from statistical analysis can be wrong.

A *type I error* is a *false positive*. In other words, we have been led to reject the null hypothesis and accept that there is a difference between two groups, when in reality one does not actually exist.

A *type II error* is a *false negative*. In other words, we have not rejected the null hypothesis, when in reality a genuine difference does exist.

Q. What do sensitivity and specificity mean?

The *sensitivity* of a test is its ability to correctly identify those people who truly have the disease. It can be calculated by the equation:

$$\frac{\text{Number of persons with the disease detected by the screening test}}{\text{Total number of tested persons with the disease}} \times 100$$

The *specificity* of a test is its ability to correctly identify those individuals who do *not* have the disease. It can be calculated by the equation:

$$\frac{\text{Number of persons without the disease who are negative to the screening test}}{\text{Total number of tested persons without the disease}} \times 100$$

Q. How does error differ from bias?

Bias refers to systematic inaccuracy due to consistent over- or under-recording. This is usually due to recorder bias, which may be subconscious.
Error is any random source of inaccuracy at any stage of a study. For example, error in collecting variables merely leads to a less precise estimate of the value (in contrast with bias). Error, because of its random nature, can usually be tackled by calculating it with appropriate statistical tests or simply by increasing the study size. Bias is a much more troublesome source of inaccuracy as its magnitude cannot really be estimated. If discovered, removing bias is difficult and usually requires fundamental alteration of the study, notably the way data are collected. However, by its nature, it often goes unrecognised, leading to erroneous conclusions.

Q. What statistical tests have you found most useful?

I have found the Student's *t*-test and the chi-squared test (χ^2-test) most useful.

Q. Tell me about t-tests.

t-tests are a commonly used statistical tool in various situations. (They were initially devised by W.S. Gosset in 1908 under the pseudonym 'Student' and they are sometimes referred to as 'Student's *t*-test'.) They require the assumption of a normal distribution and have been specifically devised to handle small samples. *t*-tests assume a null hypothesis and are used to attempt to disprove this.

They are often used where the mean and standard deviations of two samples are known and are applied to see if there is a significant difference between the sample means (unpaired *t*-test). They may also be used for paired or matched samples (paired *t-test*).

Q. Tell me about the chi-squared test.

The chi-squared test is used to assess whether an observed distribution accords with that expected, either on the basis of knowledge of the true population or on theoretical grounds. For example, if I was investigating a school with 356 boys and I found that of the 125 who lived on a housing estate with marked social deprivation, 36 had asthma, whereas of the 231 who lived elsewhere, only 44 had asthma, I could use the chi-squared test to see if this is a significant difference.

It is important to remember that chi-squared tests may only be carried out on actual numbers of occurrences and not on percentages, proportions or means of observations, or other derived statistics. In addition, the chi-squared test does not require the assumption of a normal distribution.

Q. What do you understand by the terms 'correlation' and 'regression'?

Correlation is the process of relating two quantitative variables (e.g. peak flow against height). I would do this by plotting the peak flow against the height for every individual studied. This produces a scatter diagram, which will give a visual impression of any linear association between the two variables. Calculating the *correlation coefficient* would enable me to measure the strength of the linear association mathematically. This has a value between +1, which would indicate a perfect direct relationship and −1, which would indicate a perfect inverse relationship. A value at or around zero indicates no association.

Regression, by contrast, is a predictive process. Once a scatter diagram has been obtained for two such variables, the process of linear regression would allow me to draw the line of best fit. This would then enable me to predict the value of one of the variables for a given value of the other.

The two processes are complementary. Linear regression merely allows prediction of a variable from a given set of results but it does not indicate how likely that value is in reality. This is why we need the correlation coefficient since a high value (either + or -) suggests that there probably is an association and so the regression is credible.

Q. What do you know about confidence intervals?

Confidence intervals define a range within which a given population parameter is likely to lie with a certain degree of certainty. The population parameter usually analysed is the mean and its confidence intervals are calculated from the sample mean and its standard error. In practice, a 95% confidence interval is often chosen.

Confidence intervals are based on the concept of predicting the results that we would obtain were we to repeat the study several times. Thus, if the study were to be repeated 100 times, of the 100 resulting confidence intervals, we would expect 95 of these to include the population mean.

Q. What are the advantages of using confidence intervals rather than *P*-values?

Simple statements in papers such as $P<0.05$ convey very little information about the results obtained from a study and create a rather artificial divide between 'significant' and 'non-significant'. Significance relates purely to statistical significance which may not necessarily be ideal in the context of clinical studies. Confidence intervals convey information about the magnitude of results obtained in a study, together with an estimate of the precision with which a statistic estimates a population value. This is clearly very useful information for the reader and I have noticed that an increasing number of published articles report their findings using confidence intervals rather than tests of statistical significance.

Q. What do you know about the odds ratio?

The odds ratio is the ratio of the odds of an event occurring in an experimental group (intervention/exposed to treatment) to the odds of the event occurring in a control group (not exposed to treatment). An odds ratio of 1 indicates no difference between the two groups and an odds ratio of < 1 indicates that the intervention was effective in reducing the risk of the studied outcome. It is simple to calculate and can be easily linked to other statistical tests, such as logistic regression.

Tip

● There is no way of avoiding statistics these days and unfortunately the majority of examiners now have at least a working knowledge of the most commonly used tests.

Q. What do you understand by audit?

Audit is a process by which health professionals *assess, evaluate and improve the care of patients* in a systematic way. The 1989 Department of Health White Paper *Working for Patients* was issued as part of the Government's NHS reforms and has led to the widespread mandatory use of audit within the profession. It defined medical audit as 'the systematic critical analysis of the quality of medical care, including the procedures used for diagnosis and treatment, the use of resources and the resulting outcome and quality of life for the patient'.

The audit process is best summarised by the *audit cycle*:

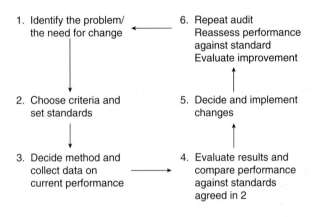

1. Identify the problem/ the need for change

2. Choose criteria and set standards

3. Decide method and collect data on current performance

4. Evaluate results and compare performance against standards agreed in 2

5. Decide and implement changes

6. Repeat audit Reassess performance against standard Evaluate improvement

Audit is therefore about self-improvement through standard-setting and so implies change as well as measurement. Broadly speaking, there are audits of *process* (investigating records to see how patients are being managed) and audits of *outcome* (investigating the results of management such as mortality and morbidity figures).

Audit may involve periodic review of recorded data (such as case notes); analysis of outcome data (such as perinatal mortality, hospital discharges or postmortem results); or collection of previously unrecorded data (such as patient satisfaction or assessment of patient education, e.g. in diabetes).

I have been involved in an audit project that was undertaken because of concern about children with acute asthma attending our A&E department waiting too long to receive their initial treatment. After discussion with the paediatric and A&E consultants, I set our standards for maximum waiting times and then measured actual performance by analysing all affected children attending A&E over a 3-month period. When comparing the two I was not surprised to find that we were only meeting our standards in 56% of cases. I presented my audit findings to those clinicians involved in the care of children with asthma in the emergency department. Following this, improvements were initiated and a repeat audit 3 months later revealed that 92% of

267

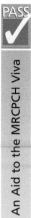

acute asthmatics received their initial asthma treatment within the maximum waiting time.

Tip

● It demonstrates both enthusiasm and wide experience if you can talk about an audit project that you have actually done, or been involved with.

SCREENING

Q. What makes a useful screening test?

When we talk about screening tests, we mean testing a whole population for a particular disease or condition. The World Health Organisation has suggested some criteria to consider when assessing the value of a screening test:

1. The *disease* or condition should:

   — be important
   — have a natural history which we understand
   — have an early asymptomatic stage
   — have agreed indications for treatment
   — have an acceptable and effective treatment

2. The *screening test* should be:

   — acceptable
   — repeatable
   — sensitive
   — specific
   — simple
   — cost-effective

Q. What do you mean by the term 'sensitive'?

Sensitivity is an indication of how good the test is at picking up people with the condition being screened for. It is also known as *the true-positive rate* and can be calculated by comparing the true-positive results with the sum of the true-positive and false-negative results:

$$\frac{\text{True-positives}}{\text{True-positives} + \text{False-negatives}}$$

In other words, sensitivity looks at the number of people correctly picked up out of all of those with the condition. A test with low sensitivity will miss a lot of people who have the condition.

Q. What do you mean by the term 'specificity'?

Specificity is an indication of how good the test is at excluding those people who do *not* have the condition being screened for. It is also known as *the true-negative rate* and can be calculated by comparing the true-negative results with the sum of the true-negative and false-positive results:

$$\frac{\text{True-negatives}}{\text{True-negatives} + \text{False-positives}}$$

In other words, specificity looks at the number of people that the test showed correctly not to have the condition out of all of those who do not have the condition. A test that has low specificity will not exclude those who have the condition and can cause a lot of anxiety.

Q. Can you think of a screening test used currently that has been successful?

All infants are currently screened for hypothyroidism by checking thyroid stimulating hormone (TSH) on a dried blood spot (collected on a Guthrie card) at the age of 5–7 days. Congenital hypothyroidism is common, with an incidence of 1 in 3500. It is usually a result of absent thyroid tissue, although it can be due to dyshormonogenesis. It is important because, if untreated, the child will have intellectual and developmental impairment. The early manifestations are non-specific and the condition may be unrecognised for several months. There is a simple and effective treatment, thyroxine, which has been agreed to be effective when started early and which prevents intellectual deterioration and growth delay.

The screening test is simple, acceptable to parents, and easily repeatable. It is cost-effective, as delaying treatment would have implications for education and independent living later in life. It is a sensitive test, picking up the majority of infants with congenital hypothyroidism, although it will miss the rare infants who are hypothyroid as a result of hypopituitarism, who will have a low TSH. It is fairly specific, but will have some false-positive results, because TSH is often slightly high in the newborn period. Repeating thyroid tests in these children as soon as the initial result is known will easily exclude those with false-positive results.

Q. What do you think of the idea of screening for medium-chain acyl-CoA dehydrogenase deficiency?

Medium-chain acyl-CoA dehydrogenase deficiency (MCAD) causes defective fatty acid oxidation. This is a serious disease, which has a high rate of morbidity and mortality as a result of inadequate energy production during periods of fasting or illness. Infants are normal on examination at birth and remain asymptomatic until they become hypoglycaemic or develop an infection. Some may present as a sudden infant death. Therefore, a screening test would fulfil the disease criteria of an important disease with an understood natural history which has a latent or asymptomatic period. Metabolic decompensation can be prevented once the diagnosis has been made by ensuring that regular fluids with high carbohydrate content are given during infection or anorexia. Carnitine abnormalities can be detected on the dried blood spot at 7 days of life.

It is also possible to screen for the majority of inborn errors of metabolism using *tandem mass spectrometry*. Further studies on the use of this method may need to be done to assess its value as a screening test, as its sensitivity, specificity and cost-effectiveness have not been established.

REFERENCE
Seashore M R 1998 Tandem spectrometry in newborn screening. Curr Opin Pediatr 10: 609–614

Miscellaneous

CRITICAL APPRAISAL OF RESEARCH PAPERS

Q. What factors go through your mind when assessing the quality of a research paper?

It is important to be able to critically appraise research papers in order to decide whether the findings can be applied in a clinical situation. There are various checklists designed to help when assessing papers relating to trials, systematic reviews, qualitative research and economic analyses. I am most familiar with assessing clinical trials of treatment options, but similar criteria can be used for any paper.

My assessment of research papers is based on three main questions:

1. Are the results valid?
2. What are the results?
3. Do the results apply to my patient group?

After reading through the paper, I apply each question in turn.

The validity of the results can be appraised mainly by looking at the methods section. Firstly, I assess whether the researchers address a clearly focused question in terms of their intervention and the outcomes considered. It is easy then to consider whether the question has clinical relevance. I check that, apart from the intervention being studied, all subjects had the same management and similar characteristics at the beginning of the trial. In a trial of a treatment, I would ascertain whether the subjects were properly randomised to treatment groups and then treated according to randomisation. This would help to eliminate bias, for example where a young group of patients might expect to have a better outcome than an elderly group, regardless of treatment. I check whether the patients and researchers were 'blinded' to the intervention, as it is very difficult for the subject or researcher not to be influenced by knowledge of their treatment.

I ensure that all patients entered into the trial are accounted for at the end of the trial and were analysed in their original groups. Finally, I look to see whether the statistical methods used were appropriate for the analysis. There are numerous statistical tests and I am not familiar with the details of all of them, but I check that simple tests of significance have been used and that parametric tests are used for data with a normal distribution. I am suspicious of the use of obscure statistical tests as this may mean that simple tests did not prove what the researchers had hoped!

When assessing *the meaning of the results*, I look for the size of the treatment effect. This will depend on the outcome measured and the number of subjects studied. The researcher should have identified how many subjects were required to give the study the power to obtain a statistically significant result before embarking on their research and this is usually published in the paper. I also check the precision of the results in terms of confidence intervals.

Although the results may reach statistical significance, I would consider whether the difference between groups is of any clinical significance.

When I decide on *the application of the results* to our patient population, I consider whether our patients have similar baseline characteristics to the trial population and whether any differences would be expected to affect the outcome of a given intervention. For example, if the trial subjects had been selected from a specialist clinic, might they have a more severe form of the condition than our patients? I check whether all clinically important outcomes were measured. If they were not, are the missing outcomes of importance to my patients? Most importantly, I assess whether the researchers have commented on any harmful effects of the treatment.

Having assessed the paper, I decide whether the findings make any difference to my clinical practice. It is easy to be critical of papers and not many seem to reach the 'gold standard', particularly in paediatric studies where the numbers studied are often small and don't have the 'power' to reach statistical significance. However, it is usually possible to assess the importance of a treatment or at least identify where further research is needed.

Tips

● You are unlikely to pass or fail on a question like this, but you may have the chance to 'win' some extra points if you demonstrate some expertise.

● Non-statisticians should avoid mentioning any specific statistical tests, just in case they are asked for more detail!

Recent developments and controversies

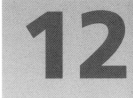

12

MMR, CROHN'S DISEASE, AND AUTISM

Q. What do you think about the suggested link between MMR vaccination, autism, and inflammatory bowel disease?

Vaccination against mumps, measles and rubella was introduced as part of the routine immunisation schedule in 1988. There have been studies from the United Kingdom, which have suggested a causal link between the combined MMR vaccine and both autism and inflammatory bowel disease.

A case series reported an increasing incidence of disorders of the *autism* spectrum and that this might be related to MMR vaccination, as the symptoms of autism were often noted soon after the vaccination had been given. However, a larger study this year was unable to establish a link between immunisation and autism. The rate of autism in children who had not been immunised was the same as in those who had. The same study also showed that although there has been a steadily increasing incidence of autism disorders, this has not changed in a stepwise manner since the introduction of MMR vaccination. The increasing incidence may be partly due to better recognition of these disorders, especially in those children with higher function. The timing of the vaccine was not found to affect the timing of onset of symptoms and signs of autism, typically noted at the age of 18–24 months.

The evidence relating to the link between MMR and *inflammatory bowel disease* is also controversial. A study comparing children who had been given measles vaccine with those who had not, showed an increased incidence of Crohn's disease. This generated interest in a causal link, but the study was criticised for poor methodology, in particular the use of unmatched controls. A study in which matched controls were used showed no increase in risk of inflammatory bowel disease. There was also a study that showed that measles virus had been identified in gut tissue affected by inflammatory bowel disease. However, it has not been possible to reproduce these findings using specific molecular biology techniques.

275

Unfortunately, the studies showing possible links with these disorders generated widespread media attention, which has led to a drop in the uptake of MMR vaccination. Studies contradicting the hypothetical connections have not been reported in the same way and there is likely to be an increase in the number of cases of mumps, measles and rubella as pool immunity drops. There is always public concern about the adverse effects of immunisation and I am frequently asked for advice about immunisations in the clinic situation. Restoring public confidence in our immunisation schedule is likely to be difficult.

Tip

● Controversial topics should always be handled with care in a viva situation. Remember that the examiner might have been in the research team that discovered the finding you are so aggressively dismissing!

REFERENCE
Wakefield A J, Murch S H, Anthony A et al 1998 Ileal lymphoid nodular hyperplasia, non-specific colitis and pervasive developmental disorder in children. Lancet 351: 637–641

SUDDEN INFANT DEATH SYNDROME

Q. Can you tell us the cause of sudden infant death syndrome?

Sudden infant death syndrome (SIDS) can be defined as the sudden and unexpected death of an infant for which, even after a thorough postmortem examination, no cause can be found. Therefore, by definition, the cause of SIDS is unknown, but we do know that there are factors related to an *increased risk* of sudden infant death. For example, there is an increased risk in multiple births and in low birth weight infants. Observational studies have shown that it is more common in those infants who sleep prone, have smokers as parents, and sleep in a bed with their parents.

Recent studies have suggested a link between *Helicobacter pylori* and SIDS. This idea started as a result of epidemiological evidence, i.e. SIDS is more common in poor communities where overcrowding is a problem and infections are more easily transmitted. A study then found more positive tests for *Helicobacter pylori* in the stomach and trachea of cases of SIDS compared with controls, using DNA extracted from tissues taken at postmortem. However, *H. pylori* infection is common in children during the first year of life and prospective data should be collected in large numbers before the link is proven.

The incidence of SIDS is currently falling, which may be partly due to the 'back to sleep' campaign of the early 1990s, in which a health education campaign encouraged families to lay their infants supine. However, the reduction in SIDS began before this campaign and may be a result of our increasing awareness of other causes of sudden infant death.

Q. Can you give us some examples of other causes of sudden infant death?

Unexpected death caused by cardiac disorders is rare in infancy, but may explain a small number of early deaths. *Re- entry supraventricular tachycardia* may be difficult to recognise clinically, but the infant is usually unwell with signs of poor feeding or breathlessness related to heart failure. *Ventricular arrhythmias* are extremely rare in infancy, but may cause unexpected death. There is disputed evidence that *QT interval prolongation* is implicated in sudden infant death. One study examined ECGs in 33 000 healthy infants at a few days of age, and then followed them for a year. The incidence of SIDS was 0.7/1000 in this cohort of patients. Half of the infants who died had a longer QT interval, corrected for heart rate, than the 97.5th% for the study group as a whole. Prolongation of the QT interval is thought to reduce cardiac stability and allows the development of ventricular fibrillation.

Other causes of death recognised more recently, which could have been defined as SIDS in the past, include metabolic disorders, particularly the *oxidation defects*, medium-chain acyl CoA and long-chain 3–hydroxyacyl CoA dehydrogenase deficiencies. These infants may deteriorate suddenly, with little preceding history of ill health, particularly after a period of relative starvation, when they are unable to utilise an alternative source of energy. Taking samples of urine and skin biopsies from infants who are brought in following unexplained death may help to pinpoint a diagnosis, which can be useful in terms of counselling the family, not only regarding the cause of their child's death but also on the risk to subsequent infants.

Finally, an unknown proportion of sudden infant deaths are a result of *direct harm by parents*. There should be suspicion about this diagnosis in families where there have been previous infant deaths, although this could equally be an indicator of inherited metabolic disorders. There may be no signs of external injury and even a postmortem may reveal no obvious cause of death, particularly if the child has been smothered.

REFERENCES

Kerr J R, Al-Khattaf A, Barson A J, Burnie J P 2000 An association between sudden infant death syndrome (SIDS) and *Helicobacter pylori* infection. Arch Dis Child 83: 429–434

Schwartz P J, Stramba-Dadiale M, Segantani A et al 1998 Prolongation of the QT interval and the sudden infant death syndrome. N Engl J of Med 338: 1709–1714

Meadow R 1999 Unnatural sudden infant death. Arch Dis Child 80: 7–14

REPORTING TO THE CORONER

Q. Tell us when you would report the death of a child to the coroner.

Section 22 of the Births and Deaths Registration Act of 1953 states that the registered medical practitioner attending the dead person during their last illness should sign the cause of death medical certificate. It is a legal requirement that this doctor has seen and examined the body after death. It is also their responsibility that the Registrar of births, deaths and marriages receives the completed certificate within 7 days of the death, even if they hand the certificate over to a third party (e.g. the parents of the dead child) to deliver it.

The attending doctor should not complete the death certificate if they have concerns about the cause of death or if certain conditions apply:

— unexplained death
— suspicious death
— death which has occurred during an operation or before recovery from the effects of the anaesthetic
— unnatural deaths or death in which violence or neglect have occurred
— abortions
— deaths where the deceased has not been seen by a medical practitioner in the 2 weeks prior to death
— all deaths occurring in custody (!)
— deaths from industrial disease or poisoning (!)

In any situation where the cause of death is not straightforward, it is worthwhile discussing the case with the coroner's office. They may well say that there is no problem and advise that the certificate can be completed by the attending medical practitioner. In more complicated cases the coroner's office will discuss with the Coroner about further action and in the meantime the certificate should not be completed. Essentially, the safest approach is to discuss any cases you are unsure of with the coroner's office so that the onus of responsibility is transferred. In Scotland such deaths should be reported to the Procurator-fiscal.

Tips

- This is a common sense question and answer. Every medical practitioner involved in writing death certificates should fully understand when they may, and may not, legally do so.

- There are different death certificates for infants dying within the first 28 days of life (form 65) and infants and children over 28 days of age (form 66).

PASS
✓

THE FETAL ORIGIN OF ADULT DISEASE

Q. Have you heard of the 'Barker' hypothesis of adult disease arising from fetal circumstances?

In the past decade the fetal origin of adult disease has emerged as a compelling hypothesis from epidemiological studies across the world. A number of adult diseases are thought to have their origins in utero, as a result of abnormal programming and adaptation by the fetus to under-or altered nutrition. Postnatal influences such as low socioeconomic status and smoking may simply compound the individual's risk of disease, rather than causing it. Nutritional insufficiency in utero may alter short-term growth but, more importantly, nutrients may be critical signals acting on 'receptors' in sensitive tissues for long-term programming of later function. The process by which this 'memory' is 'stored' may be adaptive effects on gene expression transmitted to the progeny of the originally programmed cells. Alternatively, differential cellular proliferation may alter the quantity or proportion of cell populations in a tissue permanently from the time of the initial 'insult'.

Q. OK, give me some examples of this theory.

Coronary heart disease
Disproportionate growth retardation is relatively more common in the developed world than in the underdeveloped world. Similarly, coronary heart disease (CHD) is more common in developed countries. The highest mortality from CHD is seen in men who were thin at birth and in infancy but then demonstrated accelerated weight gain in childhood, i.e. have had excellent catch up. Adaptation to fetal undernutrition by alteration of insulin sensitivity in utero may explain these findings and is supported by the finding of an increased incidence of glucose intolerance in adults who were lean at birth. Hypertension and stroke are similarly associated with thinness at birth.

Ovarian and breast cancer
Breast and ovarian cancers have been linked to high birth weight and increased weight at 12 months of age respectively. Alteration of fetal circulating oestrogen levels and patterns of gonadotrophin secretion have been implicated. Gonadotrophin release may be imprinted in utero by hormonal or nutritional influences.

Early menopause
Early menopause is correlated with shortness at birth. Sustained undernutrition in utero will cause differential nutritional supply to essential and less important organs. Primordial follicle development is maximal in the 7th month of gestation and so undernutrition in later pregnancy may result in a

smaller number of follicles being made. Menopause may then occur earlier in adult life as follicular numbers fall below a critical level.

Miscellaneous

Many other adult diseases are thought to have their origins in utero, including chronic bronchitis from impaired lung growth in utero and infancy; non-insulin-dependent diabetes mellitus; obesity; prostate cancer; subfertility in males; and ageing.

The concept of the 'fetal origins hypothesis' proposed by Barker highlights the necessity for a better understanding of fetal and infant nutrition and their long-term effects. Animal studies on nutritional manipulation, even for brief periods at critical times in development, have demonstrated long-term effects on health and growth to support this concept. It must be appreciated, however, that epidemiological 'evidence' for nutritional programming provides hypotheses rather than nutritional proof, and long-term prospective studies are required to substantiate the findings.

Tip

● Every other week there seems to be an article in the *British Medical Journal* or *Lancet* relating some anthropametric characteristic at birth and a specific adult disease. It makes one wonder if there is a particular characteristic at birth (or on entry to the paediatric profession) associated with success or failure at MRCPCH part 2 examinations! It would save an almighty amount of time, effort, and money knowing this beforehand and *must* be worthy of an MD research project after you do pass the examination (which of course you will, having read this book!).

REFERENCE
Barker D J P 1998 Mothers, babies and health in later life. 2nd edn. Churchill Livingstone, Edinburgh

MOLECULAR BIOLOGY

Q. What can you tell us about the use of molecular biology techniques in clinical practice?

Techniques in molecular biology have become increasingly sophisticated in recent years with many uses in clinical medicine, particularly in terms of detection of disease and genetic disorders.

An example of a technique that has become extremely valuable in recent clinical practice is the *polymerase chain reaction (PCR)*. PCR is a technique used to amplify specific sequences from small amounts of DNA. It can be used to demonstrate the presence or absence of a particular DNA sequence, for example the presence of DNA from meningococcus in a blood sample from a child suspected of having meningococcal infection.

The technique uses the enzyme DNA polymerase, which catalyses the formation of new strands of DNA from a mixture of complementary nucleic acid sequences, when added to a solution containing the DNA sequence being searched for. A 'primer' (that is a strand of DNA which complements a section of DNA close to the target region) and DNA polymerase are added to the mixture of nucleic acids. The DNA in the blood sample is copied to form a template, leading to formation of a piece of double stranded DNA. This is separated into two single strands by intense heat. The single strands both act as a template if more primers, which flank the target DNA sequence to be amplified, are added in excess once the solution has cooled. This cycle of primer annealing, DNA synthesis and denaturation can be repeated, resulting in an exponential increase in the amount of the required piece of DNA. The sample is then analysed by gel electrophoresis, which will show whether the target DNA is present in the original blood sample.

The polymerase chain reaction is an extremely sensitive technique, which means that even if one molecule of DNA contaminates another specimen being analysed in the laboratory, the DNA from the contaminating molecule will be amplified sufficiently to give a false-positive result.

Q. How might molecular biology help in the diagnosis of inherited disease?

When a disease is inherited, it is helpful to be able to locate the position of the gene on a chromosome. The abnormal chromosome can usually be found by studying the chromosomes from a family affected by a particular disease to find abnormalities common to the affected members of the family. Once the gene has been mapped to a chromosomal region, further localisation can be done by *linkage analysis*. This takes advantage of the fact that DNA sequences vary every few hundred bases in pairs of chromosomes, and restriction enzymes will digest strands of DNA at different places to create *restriction fragment length polymorphisms (RFLPs)*. The pattern of RFLPs can then be used

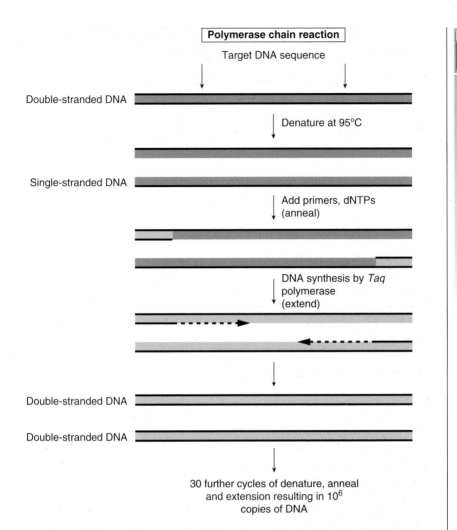

Polymerase chain reaction

Target DNA sequence

Double-stranded DNA

Denature at 95°C

Single-stranded DNA

Add primers, dNTPs
(anneal)

DNA synthesis by *Taq*
polymerase
(extend)

Double-stranded DNA

Double-stranded DNA

30 further cycles of denature, anneal
and extension resulting in 10^6
copies of DNA

as markers of disease, because the affected members of the family will share the same fragment pattern.

When the identity of a gene abnormality causing disease is known, it can be detected in the blood, or chorionic villus sample antenatally, by the polymerase chain reaction. These techniques can now be used for the diagnosis of common diseases, such as cystic fibrosis, in which 90% of gene mutations can now be detected. This can be important for confirmation of the diagnosis in a child with symptoms or for the detection of cases antenatally, so that early treatment or termination of pregnancy can be offered.

Glossary

As far as possible, you should avoid abbreviations in the viva as this tends to make you sound flippant. However, we have used some of the commoner ones to reduce the volume of the text.

ADH	Antidiuretic hormone
AIDS	Acquired immunodeficiency syndrome
ALL:	Acute lymphocytic leukaemia
AML:	Acute myeloid leukaemia
ANF:	Antinuclear factor
APLS:	Advanced paediatric life support
ARDS:	Acute respiratory distress syndrome
ASD	Atrial septal defect
ASOT:	Antistreptolysin-O titre
AXR:	Abdominal X-ray
BCG:	Bacille Calmette-Guerin
b.p.m.	beats per minute
BP	Blood pressure
CAH	Congenital adrenal hyperplasia
CHD	Congenital heart disease
CMV	Cytomegalovirus
CPK:	Creatinine phosphokinase
CPR:	Cardiopulmonary resuscitation
CRP:	C-reactive protein (?cross-reacting protein)
CT	Computerised tomography (scan)
CXR	Chest X-ray
DDAVP:	Desmopressin acetate
DHCC	Dihydroxycholecalciferol
DIC	Disseminated intravascular coagulation
DKA	Diabetic ketoacidosis
DNA	Deoxyribonucleic acid
EBV	Epstein-Barr virus
ECG	Electrocardiogram
ECMO	Extracorporeal membranous oxygenation
EDTA:	Ethylene diamine tetra acetate
EEG	Electroencephalogram
ENT	Ear, nose and throat
ESR	Erythrocyte sedimentation rate
FBC	Full blood count
FFP:	Fresh frozen plasma
G6PD:	Glucose-6-phosphate dehydrogenase

GABA:	Gamma-aminobutyric acid
GFR	Glomerular filtration rate
GOR(D):	Gastro-oesophageal reflux (disease)
HAS:	Human albumin solution
HFOV:	High frequency oscillation ventilation
HIE	Hypoxic ischaemic encephalopathy
HIV	Human immunodeficiency virus
HSP:	Henoch-Schönlein purpura
HUS:	Haemolytic uraemic syndrome
INR	International normalised ratio (for prothrombin time)
IPPV:	Intermittent positive-pressure ventilation
IQ	Intelligence quotient
ITP:	Idiopathic thrombocytopenic purpura
IVH	Intraventricular haemorrhage
LBW:	Low birth weight
LFT	Liver function tests
MMR:	Mumps, measles and rubella (vaccine)
MRI:	Magnetic resonance imaging
MRSA:	Methicillin-resistant staphylococci
NAI	Non-accidental injury
NICU:	Neonatal intensive care unit
NMDA:	N-methyl-D-aspartate
ORS:	Oral rehydration solution
PAF:	Platelet activating factor
PCR	Polymerase chain reaction
PDA	Patent ductus arteriosus
PEEP:	Positive end-expiratory pressure (ventilation)
PEFR	Peak expiratory flow rate
PET:	Positron emission tomography
PICU	Paediatric intensive care unit
PKU	Phenylketonuria
PPHN:	Persistent pulmonary hypertension of the newborn
PTH	Parathyroid hormone
PUO	Pyrexia of unknown origin
QTc:	Corrected QT (=QT/$\sqrt{RR}$ interval)
RDS	Respiratory distress syndrome
SBE:	Subacute bacterial endocarditis
SCID:	Severe combined immunodeficiency
SIADH	Syndrome of inappropriate ADH secretion
SIDS	Sudden infant death syndrome
SLE	Systemic lupus erythematosus
SPECT:	Single photon emission computed tomography
SVT	Supraventricular tachycardia
TFT:	Thyroid function test
THAM:	Trishydroxylmethylaminomethane
TORCH:	*t*oxoplasmosis, *o*ther infections, *r*ubella, *c*ytomegalovirus infection, and *h*erpes (screen)
U&E	Urea and electrolytes
URTI:	Upper respiratory tract infection
UTI	Urinary tract infection
VF:	Ventricular fibrillation
VSD	Ventricular septal defect
VT:	Ventricular tachycardia
VUR:	Vesicoureteric reflux

Index

Index